The Giants of Rheumatology

Editor

MICHAEL H. WEISMAN

RHEUMATIC DISEASE CLINICS OF NORTH AMERICA

www.rheumatic.theclinics.com

Consulting Editor
MICHAEL H. WEISMAN

February 2024 • Volume 50 • Number 1

ELSEVIER

1600 John F. Kennedy Boulevard • Suite 1800 • Philadelphia, Pennsylvania, 19103-2899
http://www.theclinics.com

RHEUMATIC DISEASE CLINICS OF NORTH AMERICA Volume 50, Number 1
February 2024 ISSN 0889-857X, ISBN 13: 978-0-443-13027-4

Editor: Joanna Gascoine
Developmental Editor: Isha Singh

Rheumatic Disease Clinics of North America (ISSN 0889-857X) is published quarterly by Elsevier Inc., 360 Park Avenue South, New York, NY 10010-1710. Months of issue are February, May, August, and November. Business and editorial offices: 1600 John F. Kennedy Boulevard, Suite 1800, Philadelphia, PA 19103-2899. Periodicals postage paid at New York, NY and additional mailing offices. Subscription prices are USD 384.00 per year for US individuals, USD 100.00 per year for US students and residents, USD 449.00 per year for Canadian individuals, USD 100.00 per year for Canadian students/residents, USD 489.00 per year for international individuals, and USD 230.00 per year for foreign students/residents. For institutional access pricing please contact Customer Service via the contact information below. To receive student/resident rate, orders must be accompanied by name of affiliated institution, date of term, and the *signature* of program/residency coordinator on institution letterhead. Orders will be billed at individual rate until proof of status received. Foreign air speed delivery is included in all *Clinics* subscription prices. All prices are subject to change without notice. **POSTMASTER:** Send address changes to *Rheumatic Disease Clinics of North America,* Elsevier Health Sciences Division, Subscription Customer Service, 3251 Riverport Lane, Maryland Heights, MO 63043. **Customer Service: 1-800-654-2452 (US and Canada). From outside of the US and Canada: 314-447-8871. Fax: 314-447-8029. For print support, e-mail: JournalsCustomerService-usa@elsevier.com. For online support, e-mail: JournalsOnlineSupport-usa@elsevier.com.**

Reprints. For copies of 100 or more of articles in this publication, please contact the Commercial Reprints Department, Elsevier Inc., 360 Park Avenue South, New York, New York, 10010-1710; Tel.: +1-212-633-3874, Fax: +1-212-633-3820, and E-mail: reprints@elsevier.com.

Rheumatic Disease Clinics of North America is covered in *MEDLINE/PubMed (Index Medicus), Current Contents/Clinical Medicine, Science Citation Index, ISI/BIOMED,* and *EMBASE/Excerpta Medica.*

Contributors

CONSULTING EDITOR

MICHAEL H. WEISMAN, MD
Adjunct Professor of Medicine, Stanford University, Distinguished Professor of Medicine Emeritus, David Geffen School of Medicine at UCLA, Professor of Medicine Emeritus, Cedars-Sinai Medical Center, Los Angeles, California, USA

EDITOR

MICHAEL H. WEISMAN, MD
Adjunct Professor of Medicine, Stanford University, Distinguished Professor of Medicine Emeritus, David Geffen School of Medicine at UCLA, Professor of Medicine Emeritus, Cedars-Sinai Medical Center, Los Angeles, California, USA

AUTHORS

DANIEL A. ALBERT, MD, MACR
Professor of Medicine and Pediatrics, Division of Rheumatology, Dartmouth Hitchcock Medical Center, Lebanon, New Hampshire, USA

DANIEL G. BAKER, MD
CEO, Kira Biotech Pty Ltd, Fortitude Valley, Queensland, Australia

JOSHUA F. BAKER, MD, MSCE
Associate Professor of Medicine (Rheumatology), Hospital of the University of Pennsylvania and the Veteran's Administration Medical Center, Instructor in Medicine, University of Pennsylvania, Perelman School of Medicine, Director, Clinical Research Center, Corporal Michael J. Crescenz VA Medical Center, Philadelphia, Pennsylvania, USA

S. LOUIS BRIDGES Jr, MD, PhD
Physician-in-Chief and Chair, Department of Medicine, Franchellie M. Cadwell Professor of Medicine, Chief, Division of Rheumatology, Hospital for Special Surgery, Chief, Division of Rheumatology, Joseph P. Routh Professor of Rheumatic Diseases in Medicine, Weill Cornell Medicine, Weill Cornell Medical College, New York, New York, USA

GRANT W. CANNON, MD
Emeritus Professor of Medicine, Division of Rheumatology, University of Utah School of Medicine, Salt Lake City, Utah, USA

DANIEL O. CLEGG, MD
Emeritus Professor of Medicine, Division of Rheumatology, University of Utah School of Medicine, Salt Lake City, Utah, USA

MARY E. CSUKA, MD
Professor of Medicine, Division of Rheumatology, Department of Medicine, Medical
College of Wisconsin, Milwaukee, Wisconsin, USA

MARY K. CROW, MD
Professor, Mary Kirkland Center for Lupus Research, Hospital for Special Surgery,
SSRUU, New York, New York, USA

STEFFEN GAY, MD
Professor Emeritus, Senior Consultant, Department of Rheumatology, University Hospital
Zürich, Switzerland

PAUL HALVERSON, MD
Emeritus Professor of Medicine, Division of Rheumatology, Department of Medicine,
Medical College of Wisconsin, Milwaukee, Wisconsin, USA

MARC C. HOCHBERG, MD, MPH, MACP, MACR
Professor of Medicine and Epidemiology and Public Health, Head, Division of
Rheumatology and Clinical Immunology, Vice Chair, Department of Medicine, University
of Maryland School of Medicine, Director, Medical Care Clinical Center, Veterans Affairs
Maryland Health Care System, Baltimore, Maryland, USA

JONATHAN KAY, MD
Division of Rheumatology, Department of Medicine, UMass Chan Medical School, UMass
Memorial Medical Center, Worcester, Massachusetts, USA

EDWARD R. LEW, BA
Department of Political Science and Legal Studies, University of Massachusetts Amherst

MATTHEW H. LIANG, MD, MPH
Professor of Medicine, Harvard Medical School, Professor of Health Policy and
Management, Harvard TH Chan School of Public Health, Section of Rheumatology,
Boston VA Healthcare System, Division of Rheumatology, Inflammation, and Immunity,
Brigham and Women's Hospital, Boston, Massachusetts, USA

JAMES S. LOUIE, MD, MACR, FACP
Professor Emeritus, Rheumatology and Arthritis, UCLA, Los Angeles, California, USA

THOMAS A. MEDSGER, MD
Emeritus Professor, University of Pittsburgh School of Medicine, Pittsburgh,
Pennsylvania, USA

MICHELLE A. PETRI, MD, MPH
Division of Rheumatology, Department of Medicine, Johns Hopkins School of Medicine,
Baltimore, Maryland, USA

ROSS E. PETTY, CM, MD, PhD, FRCPC, ScD (Hon)
Emeritus Professor of Pediatric Rheumatology, University of British Columbia, Vancouver,
Canada

ANTHONY M. REGINATO, PhD, MD
Division of Rheumatology, Departments of Medicine and Dermatology, Rhode Island
Hospital, Warren Alpert Medical School of Brown University, Providence, Rhode Island,
USA

WILLIAM NEAL ROBERTS Jr, MD
Professor of Medicine, Division of Rheumatology, University of Kentucky Medical Center,
Lexington, Kentucky, USA

ANN K. ROSENTHAL, MD
Will and Cava Ross Professor of Medicine, Chief of Rheumatology, Rheumatology Division, Medical College of Wisconsin, Milwaukee, Wisconsin, USA

RICHARD M. SILVER, MD
Distinguished University Professor, Division of Rheumatology and Immunology, Medical University of South Carolina, Charleston, South Carolina, USA

JOSEF S. SMOLEN, MD
Handling Editor, Mary Kirkland Center for Lupus Research, Hospital for Special Surgery, New York, New York, USA

VIRGINIA D. STEEN, MD
Professor of Medicine, Georgetown University School of Medicine, Washington, DC, USA

DANIEL J. WALLACE, MD, FACP, MACR
Clinical Professor of Medicine, David Geffen School of Medicine, UCLA, Associate Director, Rheumatology Fellowship Program, Cedars-Sinai Medical Center, Los Angeles, California, USA

ARTHUR WEINSTEIN, MD, FACP, FRCP, MACR
Clinical Professor of Medicine, Loma Linda University, Loma Linda, California, USA; Clinical Professor Emeritus of Medicine, Georgetown University, Washington, DC, USA

H. JAMES WILLIAMS, MD
Emeritus Professor of Medicine, Division of Rheumatology, University of Utah School of Medicine, Salt Lake City, Utah, USA

PATRICIA WOO, CBE, FMedSci, MBBS, PhD, FRCP, FRCPCH
Emeritus Professor of Paediatric Rheumatology, University College, London, United Kingdom

Contents

us who had the opportunity to train under him have been inspired to carry it forward.

Richard M. Silver

E. Carwile LeRoy, M.D. was a pioneer in the study of systemic sclerosis (SSc, scleroderma). His early medical training was strongly influenced by notable clinical investigators including Dr Kenneth Brinkhous, Dr Charles Christian and Dr Albert Sjoerdsma. Dr LeRoy is remembered for his seminal observations on the over-production of collagen by scleroderma fibroblasts and for his vascular hypothesis on the pathogenesis of scleroderma. The Division of Rheumatology & Immunology at the Medical University of South Carolina, established by Dr LeRoy, is world renowned for its clinical and translational studies of scleroderma and has produced many of the leaders in the international scleroderma community.

Mary K. Crow and Josef S. Smolen

Dr Charles L Christian arrived in New York City in 1953, having grown up in Wichita, Kansas, and graduating from medical school at Case Western Reserve in Cleveland, Ohio. In New York, Dr Christian embarked on training in internal medicine at Columbia's Presbyterian Hospital where he met an individual who would shape the course of his career, Dr Charles Ragan, a founder of the Arthritis Foundation. Dr Christian, or Chuck as he was usually called, went on to shape the developing field of rheumatology, advancing understanding of our most complex diseases as an investigator, master clinician, mentor, and academic leader. During an era when the cellular and humoral features of the immune system were just coming into focus, Chuck performed laboratory experiments with precision and creativity to achieve new understanding of 3 significant diseases: rheumatoid arthritis, systemic lupus erythematosus, and vasculitis. Review of his publications from the 1950s and 1960s provides a window into a time when figures were hand drawn and papers often had a single author. While the tools of technology that we rely on today were not available to Chuck, his insights have had a sustained impact on how we understand and treat autoimmune rheumatic diseases. His talents and his dedication to patients, colleagues, science, and medicine supported a lifetime of remarkable contributions

S. Louis Bridges Jr. and Steffen Gay

Dr Claude Bennett provided local, national, and international leadership in rheumatology when it was developing as a subspecialty of internal medicine. His early contributions included work in helping to understand at the molecular level how antibodies are formed. Under his leadership, UAB grew into a nationally respected institution known for its high-quality clinical care, impactful research, and outstanding training programs. His many contributions have had a lasting effect on the fields of rheumatology, medicine, and immunology. Throughout his career, he served as a role model and was widely respected for his wise advice and superb mentorship.

Daniel J. Wallace

In the year 1950, Edmund Dubois was asked to evaluate eight patients who had positive results from a new blood test known as the LE cell prep. This was the springboard for him to launch a career that elucidated new and unique insights into the pathogenesis, clinical presentation, laboratory testing, and treatment of systemic lupus erythematosus. Between 1950 and 1985, he treated more than 2000 patients with the disorder and wrote the principal textbook on the subject.

James S. Louie

Carl M. Pearson was an energetic and exceptional physician–scholar-leader who founded, established, and broadened the Divisions of Rheumatology at University of California in Los Angeles (UCLA) beginning in 1956. His studies to induce myositis by injecting muscle saturated with the heat-killed tubercle bacillus, an emulsifier, and mineral oil (Freund's adjuvant) enabled his report that polyarthritis occurred with Freund's adjuvant alone in certain strains of rat and mice. This model of adjuvant arthritis allowed the next generation of studies to assess therapies for autoimmune diseases.

Anthony M. Reginato, Michelle A. Petri, and Jonathan Kay

Walter Bauer was instrumental in the development of rheumatology as a medical subspecialty, promoting careful clinical observation and description and bringing basic scientists and clinicians together to study the "anatomy, chemical composition, and metabolism of connective tissue" in the laboratory. Marian Wilkins Ropes was a pioneering woman in medicine: the first female medical resident at the Massachusetts General Hospital, the first woman appointed as an assistant professor of clinical medicine at Harvard Medical School, the first woman elected to membership in the American Society of Clinical Investigation, and the first woman elected president of the American Rheumatism Association. Both Bauer and Ropes were 'giants in rheumatology' who combined clinical observation and clinical care with basic science laboratory investigations to further the understanding of the rheumatic diseases.

Patricia Woo and Ross E. Petty

Eric Bywaters and Barbara Ansell were, without doubt, two of the giants in the field of Rheumatology. With their keen clinical observations and their visionary development of a dedicated multidisciplinary program focusing on diagnosis, treatment, and research, they are remembered as the founders of the modern specialty of Pediatric Rheumatology.

reinvented himself in population health. In contrast to reductionist laboratory-based research, his work embraced complexity and made action researchable and research action-oriented. Some innovations did not survive as originally conceived, but their ethos became mainstream. These included evidence-based management, shared physician-patient decision-making, self-management, critical evaluation of medical technology and diagnostics, and chronic disease management. Through the rise of the twentieth century American biomedical medicine, medical education, and slow-motion health care delivery crises that still occur, Holman changed the debate in a time when the funding, the people, the technology, and the need made all things seem possible.

RHEUMATIC DISEASE CLINICS OF NORTH AMERICA

SERIES OF RELATED INTEREST

Emergency Medicine Clinics
Available at: https://www.emed.theclinics.com/
Medical Clinics
Available at: https://www.medical.theclinics.com/

THE CLINICS ARE AVAILABLE ONLINE!
Access your subscription at:
www.theclinics.com

Preface

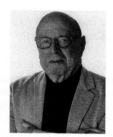

Michael H. Weisman, MD
Editor

This is both a preface and a foreword. Why? Because, as within a preface, I will speak plainly about the purpose and creation of this issue, how and why this story came into being, and what the main points are going forward. But, as within a foreword, I should tell the reader why he or she should read the issue along with its potential importance in the field. So, bear with me. From the very beginning this whole journey got started a long time ago for me when my mentor, Nathan Zvaifler, invited his senior colleagues in the field of Rheumatology to UCSD starting in the 1970s with the purpose of enriching the scholarly and academic experience of his Fellows and colleagues. He even arranged for many of these superstars to visit the other academic institutions in the area: Scripps Clinic and Research Foundation and the Balboa Navy Hospital. Maybe Nate did it because he wanted to "show off" what he could do and toot his own horn to the more established senior scientists and investigators at Scripps, but who really cares since, at the end of the day, the result was truly wonderful. For the next 20 years or so, we spent several days each year with the likes of Eric Bywaters, Dan McCarty, Gerry Rodnan, Mary Betty Stevens, Chuck Christian, and so many others. It is hard for me to tell either then or today if our Fellows and my colleagues felt the magnitude of this experience as much as I did, but there is no doubt that it created an indelible and completely life-changing set of experiences for me.

What did I learn? First, it was the absolute importance of the humility of what it means to be an expert, and furthermore, why it is so important to not only obtain that expertise but also to be able to impart that experience onto others. These people who came to visit did not get there by luck or by accident. The whole enterprise gave me the focus on what it means to be a mentor and how to transmit that mentorship to others. Can you imagine what it must have been like for a relatively naive junior person in the field to go to a national ACR meeting all alone and run into someone like Charles Christian, and he actually remembered my name and said hello! One of the interesting anecdotes from having to arrange the clinical sessions with these experts every year was the need to find interesting cases to present to them in a teaching format. The usual default tendency was to find a case that was incredibly complex and had already

Rheum Dis Clin N Am 50 (2024) xiii–xiv
https://doi.org/10.1016/j.rdc.2023.09.003
0889-857X/24/© 2023 Published by Elsevier Inc.

stumped our own experts at UCSD; what I discovered was that our visiting Professor really didn't know what to do either, so the whole discussion was useless. What I learned was that we needed to present fairly common clinical scenarios where the expert would be able to give us his or her own approach to a usual clinical dilemma. In that way, we were able to obtain the breadth and depth of their own unique experience and truly learn from a "master" clinician. This awareness has stood by me for all of my own life as a teacher and as an investigator.

Why should we do this issue today, and what could it mean to our early career colleagues as well as our students and Fellows? First, it is likely that our current trainees do not even know the names of the individuals in this issue, so at the very least these articles will fill an important void. But the real reason is likely to be that our current educational and experiential environment is on overload status whereby only immediate access to summarized data appears to be important or used at all. Fellows today read homogenized guidelines immediately available on a handheld device in order to make a diagnostic or therapeutic decision. It isn't at all clear to them where the information comes from or who or what group actually created it from scratch. Without sounding like an artificial intelligence denier, or even worse, an apologist for the "good old days"—which weren't really that good—our trainees and Fellows should know where the information they use comes from, and who did it, how it was done, and why was the question asked in the first place. What were the observations from clinical medicine that provoked those studies and for which a question need to be answered? Perhaps an exposure from our Fellows and trainees to these giants and a subsequent appreciation of the impact on our field by these pioneers, and how they thought critically and scientifically about their patients and their needs, might entice even one of them to pursue a career so wonderfully represented by these unique individuals. Wouldn't that be a nice result?

Finally, an apology and a disclaimer are in order. Clearly, this is a convenience sample of highly selected individuals who qualify for "giant" status at the very least on my behalf. Your favorite giant may not be here, and the list is neither exhaustive nor complete. The initial selection bias came from my own experience with Nate's colleagues who came to visit us at UCSD during the years starting in the mid-1970s. I tried to fill the gap of individuals who didn't visit with those men and women who clearly made their mark on our field during the same timeframe, and even beforehand. I did the best I could with our wonderful contributors and writers, alive and well today, who could remember enough to create our content. They did a marvelous job, and we learned a lot from the digging and exploring they accomplished I apologize for any omissions, but the contributors and chapter writers get all the credit for what was actually done.

Michael H. Weisman, MD
David Geffen School of Medicine at UCLA
Cedars-Sinai Medical Centers
10800 Wilshire Boulevard, #404
Los Angeles, CA 90024, USA

E-mail address:
Michael.Weisman@cshs.org

Naomi Rothfield, MD, MACR
A Giant Gift in a Small Package

Arthur Weinstein, MD, FRCP, MACR[a,b,]*

KEYWORDS

- Rheumatology • Systemic lupus erythematosus • Antinuclear antibodies
- Corticosteroids • Rothfield

INTRODUCTION

Naomi Rothfield died July 2, 2023 at age 94 (**Fig. 1–3**). With high intelligence, intellectual curiosity, drive, and New York feistiness, she propelled herself to the upper echelons of academic rheumatology from the 1950s to her retirement over 60 years later. Through it all she suffered, and overcame, the slings and arrows that professional, high-achieving women faced in the male-dominated academic culture in the United States. Not only that, but during those early years, she raised a family with 4 small children.

As an undergraduate at Bard College, she was repeatedly told that getting into medical school was almost impossible for a woman. When she applied to a number of prestigious medical schools, they wrote back that they did not take women. When she did get interviews, she was told that they had just started accepting a few women. One interviewer stated he disapproved of women in medicine, and another asked her only whether she planned on getting married and how many children she expected to have.

She was accepted by a few medical schools in New York State and graduated from New York University School of Medicine (NYU) in 1955. Her formative clinical years were spent at Lenox Hill and Bellevue Hospitals in New York City and an interest in rheumatology led to success in obtaining an Arthritis Foundation Fellowship. Interestingly, applications to do a fellowship in some of the few extant Rheumatology Centers in the United States were met with similar skepticism that she had become used to, especially when they learned that by this time she had 4 children!

However, she was accepted by Currier McEwan at NYU and was learning laboratory techniques with immunopathologist Robert McCluskey, one of the pioneers in the measurement of tissue antibodies by immunofluorescence. Those were heady days for laboratory and clinical immunology and early rheumatology at NYU with Drs McEwen, McCluskey, Morris Ziff, Ed Franklin, Gerald Weissman, and Naomi. Therefore, it was a natural evolution for her to develop an academic interest in immunology and a

[a] Loma Linda University, Loma Linda, CA, USA; [b] Georgetown University, Washington, DC, USA
* 2173 Edinboro Avenue, Claremont, CA 91711.
E-mail address: aw89@georgetown.edu

Rheum Dis Clin N Am 50 (2024) 1–5
https://doi.org/10.1016/j.rdc.2023.08.014
0889-857X/24/© 2023 Elsevier Inc. All rights reserved.
rheumatic.theclinics.com

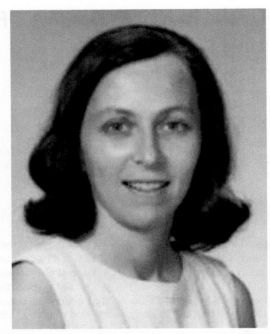

Fig. 1. Naomi Rothfield as a young trainee. (With permission from University of Connecticut.)

clinical focus on patients with systemic lupus erythematosus (SLE). She remained on the NYU faculty for 9 years after her fellowship when, in 1968, she became the first Chief of Rheumatology at a newly opened medical school, the University of Connecticut School of Medicine (UConn) in Farmington. She has remained there for the rest of her academic career until her retirement about 7 years ago. Sadly, Larry Rothfield died in December 2022. He was her husband and life partner of 69 years and was himself an eminent microbiologist and Department Chair at UConn.

SCIENTIFIC CONTRIBUTIONS

In her early publications and throughout her scientific and clinical career, Naomi's focus had been to characterize the breadth of the clinical, laboratory, and immunologic features of SLE with a view to accurate diagnosis and appropriate treatment. What may seem so well known now 60years later was so new and groundbreaking then. So much so that of her first 15 publications, 4 were in the New England Journal of Medicine, 2 in Journal of Clinical Investigation, and others in Journal of the American Medical Association (JAMA) and Arthritis & Rheumatology. Her descriptions of lupus skin disease, renal disease, children with SLE, and pregnancy in SLE were particularly noteworthy. She also had an abiding interest in the characterization and clinical significance of antinuclear antibodies (ANAs) and anti-DNA antibodies in the serum of SLE patients with many publications in highly recognized journals. Naomi also described the use of serum complement in SLE diagnosis and the association of inherited complement deficiencies with SLE, as well as the role of corticosteroids in the development of aseptic bone necrosis. She published on the appropriate use of antimalarials and corticosteroids in the treatment of SLE both in clinical studies and review articles.

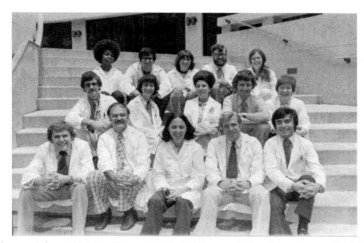

Fig. 2. Rheumatology Division UConn 1976. (With permission from Uconn Health Center.)

Her abiding scientific curiosity and interest in ANAs in autoimmune diseases translated to many clinical and laboratory studies of scleroderma-related ANAs, characterization of their nuclear targets and their clinical significance, again resulting in many publications in prestigious journals.

In order to achieve her scientific goals, Naomi had to be successful in obtaining research grants from many organizations. Most prominent were Veterans Affairs (VA) and National Institutes of Health (NIH) funding and she was Director of the NIH-supported UConn Multipurpose Arthritis Center for 20 years.

As befits, a successful academic Naomi served on many national committees of the Arthritis Foundation, the American College of Rheumatology, the Lupus Foundation of America, the NIH General Study Section A, FDA Advisory Committee, VA Immunology Committee as well editorial boards of Journal of Rheumatology, Lupus, Arthritis and Rheumatology and Clinical Immunology and immunopathology.

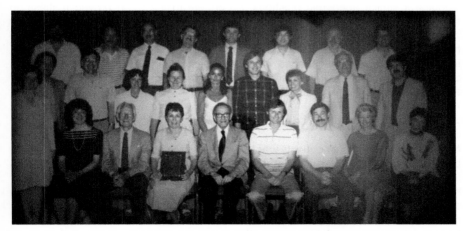

Fig. 3. Naomi with Currier McEwan, Morris Ziff, current and former UConn faculty and fellows at ACR. (With permission from University of Connecticut.)

Her academic excellence led to many guest lectureships and scientific awards including, the Pemberton Memorial Lecture from the Philadelphia Rheumatism Society, the Solomon A. Berson Medical Alumni Achievement Award in Clinical Sciences from the NYU School of Medicine, and Master, American College of Rheumatology.

COLLABORATIONS AND MENTORING

Throughout her career Naomi was an enthusiastic collaborator with many clinicians from many specialties and backgrounds, and laboratory-based scientists to help to characterize the multiplicity of clinical, pathologic, and serologic features of SLE and scleroderma. Furthermore, all the Rheumatology fellows and faculty collaborated with her in these investigations and authored and co-authored numerous publications. She was always the center and driver of the diverse investigative groups. Her fellows and faculty came from all over the country and other countries to work with her in the small community of Farmington, Connecticut, and many took back their "Naomi-acquired" skills to head up their own Lupus programs elsewhere. A number of her trainees and faculty became Rheumatology Division Chiefs in the United States, Canada, and Iceland. Naomi led by example. Her scientific curiosity and insights were outstanding and led from clinical questions at the bedside to answers, in organized observational studies and laboratory collaborations.

IMPACT ON RHEUMATOLOGY

Naomi Rothfield obviously had an important scientific impact on the evolving knowledge of clinical SLE and the role of ANAs in SLE and scleroderma. She was also a member the Committee which produced the landmark publication by the American College of Rheumatology of the Criteria for the Classification of Systemic Lupus Erythematosus. She also mentored the careers of numerous faculty and trainees who became physician scientists and practicing rheumatologists.

Her major impact in rheumatology, as the author believes, was to demonstrate that women could succeed and lead at a time when few were being given that opportunity. An example of that fight for equality happened a few years after starting at UConn. She and 2 other women faculty learned that their salary was lower than their male colleagues at similar academic positions. An appeal to the Dean proved fruitless so they went to the federal authorities as it contravened Title XIX regulations. They partially won their case, but they received only 1year's back differential pay. Naomi had constantly to prove that she could be as good as, if not better than, her male colleagues and ultimately succeeded with the recognition she received from her peers. She was, for many, a trailblazer and an example that talented women could fight for and attain positions of high academic standing.

CONTRIBUTIONS TO PATIENT CARE

Naomi's dedication to her patients was legendary. In the outpatient clinics and on hospital rounds, she was passionate and tireless in pursuit of their cure and of their comfort. Her patients were able to reach her at any time, since she provided them with her home and work numbers. In this way, she was totally involved in their medical and personal lives, in their accomplishments, and with their pregnancies and babies. Patients recognized her knowledge and dedication to their welfare, and they flocked to the small suburb of Hartford, Connecticut, from all over the northeast, enabling her to establish one of the larger lupus clinics in the country.

Naomi was also instrumental in helping to organize and establish a lupus group in Connecticut to assist lupus patients, especially newly diagnosed patients, connect with each other. She wanted them to know they were not alone and could provide knowledge and emotional support to each other. This became the Connecticut Lupus Chapter and one of the founding chapters of the Lupus Foundation of America.

SUMMARY

Naomi Rothfield was truly a pied piper of lupus. Under her leadership, numerous professionals focused their clinical and research activities to benefit lupus patients. An outstanding academic, she helped break the glass ceiling in academic rheumatology and many women have since risen the ranks of academic success.

DISCLOSURE

The author has nothing to disclose.

Nathan Zvaifler

Daniel A. Albert, MD, MACR

KEYWORDS

- Nathan Zvaifler • Complement • Rheumatoid arthritis
- University of California, San Diego • Synovitis

KEY POINTS

- Nathan Zvaifler was an innovative clinician-scientist and mentor.
- He was a dominant figure in Rheumatology in the 1970s and 1980s.
- His trainees retained his investigative spirit and went on to lead many programs across the country.
- His legacy is multidimensional as a scientist uncovering the pathogenesis of rheumatoid arthritis, as a leader in the field of rheumatology and as a mentor to legions of budding rheumatologists.

INTRODUCTION

Nathan Zvaifler was one of the most remarkable individuals that I have ever met in the field of rheumatology, but it's important to describe him within time and place, and in particular in the context of my own journey. I wonder if we will ever encounter people like Nate in the future, maybe not, but it is worth recalling them as we consider our own legacies. The best way to characterize Nate Zvaifler is to place him in the context of what rheumatology was and possibly never will be again, for better or for worse.

MY START IN RHEUMATOLOGY

When I was a medical student at New York University in the early 1970s, I attended an honors seminar hosted by Gerald Weissman, open to everyone, and we met in a fancy board room where we discussed journal articles while imbibing wine and nibbling cheese. Those were the days. Many of the articles reflected Dr Weissman's interest in immunology and inflammation. I was further stimulated by the members of the pathology department including Chandler Stetson, who had us to dinner at his elegant house in Westchester, the Nussensweigs, who made us think that science was fun and endlessly interesting, and Michael Heidelberger, who continued to make scientific contributions until he was over 100 years old. I was curious about these mysterious autoimmune diseases that they were all studying and heard about

Division of Rheumatology, Dartmouth Hitchcock Medical Center, Rheumatology 5C, Dartmouth Medical Center, 1 Medical Center Drive, Lebanon, NH 03756, USA
E-mail address: daniel.a.albert@hitchcock.org

Rheum Dis Clin N Am 50 (2024) 7–13
https://doi.org/10.1016/j.rdc.2023.08.015
0889-857X/24/© 2023 Elsevier Inc. All rights reserved.
rheumatic.theclinics.com

a book that was written for novices like myself called the *Primer of Rheumatic Diseases*. The text was issued every few years with updated material and got larger and larger, while still maintaining a focus on medical students, residents, fellows, and other trainees. I had heard about this book but never saw an actual copy. One evening I decided to track it down. I went to the laboratory building where several floors had been designated Irvington House, dedicated to the study of rheumatic fever. There I met Edward Franklin (the co-discover of Meltzer-Franklin disease, now called mixed cryoglobulinemia and heavy chain disease related to Waldenstrom's Macroglobulinemia) in the hallway, and he gave me a copy. Later I learned there was a companion slide collection made available by the American Rheumatism Association (now called the American College of Rheumatology). How could I pass up an opportunity to go into a field that made such a concerted effort to engage students in their discipline?

Suitably primed, I went to the University of North Carolina at Chapel Hill for residency in internal medicine. There I had the good fortune of being on service with 2 of the most engaging and enthusiastic attendings: Peter Utsinger and Nortin Hadler. They cemented my decision to pursue a career in rheumatology. I worked with Nortin on a variety of studies, including the first multicenter outcome study of prognostic factors in systemic lupus, reviewing microfiche of handwritten records on 200 lupus patients at Chapel Hill. Nortin and I also reviewed Marian Ropes' hand-written notes on elementary school lined paper on her patients, where she graphed their renal function, blood counts, and so forth, in order to compare her results with other life table data sets, to perform the first meta-analysis comparing the data before and after the introduction of corticosteroid therapy. I also got to meet Hal Holman, Ted Pincus, and Jim Fries through the Robert Wood Johnson (RWJ) Program and was introduced to their revolutionary use of patient-reported outcomes and chronologically documented disease variables as a tool for understanding disease patterns and responses to therapies.

FIRST ENCOUNTER WITH NATHAN ZVAIFLER

It was from these mentors that I first learned about Nathan Zvaifler. I was completing my residency and the RWJ Clinical Scholars Program when I approached Nortin and Peter about fellowship. I believe Peter knew Nate from Georgetown where Peter went to medical school. Having spent 4 delightful years in Chapel Hill (albeit a place where no one ever heard of bagel lox and cream cheese), I was ready for a new venue and wanted their opinion on where I should go. Both of them identified Nate Zvaifler as one of the smartest and most innovative thinkers in rheumatology. He had published a revolutionary theory that rheumatoid arthritis was due to immune complex deposition in the synovial cavity with complement activation and consequent inflammation (*The Journal of Clinical Investigation* 43; 1372–1382, 1964) Thus, the immune complex could take its toll in the vascular system though cryoglobulinemia and in the synovial cavity in rheumatoid arthritis. I then made the obligatory tour of the elite rheumatology programs to see if I could secure a fellowship. I went to Pittsburgh to meet with the ineffable Gerald Rodnan, who interviewed me and made an indelible impression as he slapped the desk he was sitting at to emphasize that "every rheumatologist loves the gout," a statement that no one would argue with. However, wanting to go to the West Coast my first choice was the University of California, Los Angeles (UCLA) led by Carl Pearson and a group of luminaries including Rodney Bluestone who interviewed me. In those days there was no match, and you were on your own to find a program. Dr Bluestone said they already filled their slots, but he would let me know if an additional slot became available.

The next day I traveled down the I-5 to San Diego where I interviewed at the University of California, San Diego (UCSD). I met several faculty members who were kind but noncommittal. I then went to Dr Zvaifler's house on Moonridge Drive in La Jolla that evening. The property was enclosed in a wooden fence that kept the house hidden. The gate opened to a Japanese garden and a path to the front door which crossed over a black bottom pool to the entrance of a modern glass and wood house cantilevered over the canyon with a 180-degree view of La Jolla bay. The house was an art gallery with beautiful sculptures and paintings. You met up instantly with a large Afghan hound named Hashish. I think we had drinks, but I can only remember that Dr Zvaifler (on the strength of recommendations from Nortin Hadler and Peter Utsinger) offered me a position on the spot. We shook on it, and I was elated to be going to San Diego in a great program headed by a legendary physician scientist. The next day I received a call from Dr Bluestone offering me a position at UCLA, but I declined because, although I did not sign a contract, my handshake was my word. It was one of the best decisions I have made in my life.

SAN DIEGO IN THE1970S

When I got to San Diego eager to buy a house in the booming Southern California market, I borrowed $7000 from my parents and bought a tract house in a community called Allied Gardens. The house was fine, but the previous owners had German shepherds that were infested with fleas who had abandoned their hosts and resided in the carpets. We walked into the house and were promptly attacked with such ferocity we abandoned the house for a motel until it could be tented and fumigated, which solved the situation. It was a few miles from the hospital in Mission Hills necessitating a car ride, but we were soon able to trade up to a lovely Spanish-style house in Mission Hills that was all of 900 square feet after the garage had been converted to a second bedroom. But it had a deck over a canyon with a hot tub where in the evening you could hear the monkeys in the zoo in Balboa Park and see the sunset over the Pacific Ocean, even though the ocean was out of view. From this residence, the trip to the hospital, offices, and laboratories was walkable, but I preferred to bike since the weather was almost always terrific and it was flat from the house to my destination. Once a week we went to the campus in La Jolla, but the hospital that is now there (originally called Thornton. now called Jacobs Medical Center) had not been built and my only connection to the campus was several years later when I worked in Jay Seegmiller's laboratory.

Rheumatology at University of California, San Diego

The program was the usual outpatient clinic and inpatient consultation and the volume was not excessive, but we made the most of each encounter with our stalwart attendings primarily Nate, Harry Bluestein, and Michael Weisman. Each patient was discussed in exorbitant detail and every ounce of learning was extracted. While we learned a great deal from the attendings and patients, we also had a tremendous comradery with our fellowship group. They were all close friends and colleagues to this day, most notably Chris Burns who is a fellow attending at Dartmouth, Rick Silver with whom I did residency and fellowship and took up pediatric rheumatology just out of interest and patient need, Louise Keough who stayed in San Diego as did Alan Cohen, and many others. It was an upbeat and energetic atmosphere that Nate promoted in his inimical way of quietly understating a problem but still conveying his enthusiasm for the question. He was sometimes hard to read and spoke elliptically, so you needed to think. We often had to figure out why did he say that and fill in several lines of logic that led to his statement.

Harry had just finished a sabbatical that he stayed in San Diego which was typical of Harry. He liked things to be the way they were and ascribed to the fixed heartbeat theory that you were allotted a certain number of heartbeats for your life and if you used them up you would die prematurely. He took his time away in Jay Seegmiller's laboratory studying the immunodeficiencies associated with adenosine deaminase and purine nucleoside phosphorylase deficiencies. These fascinating disorders were the topic of discussion when we spoke about my research project since Harry was the fellowship director. I decided to pursue that project and subsequently spent an extra year in Jay's laboratory. During that year I also spent 6 months doing clinic at San Diego Children's Hospital studying pediatric rheumatology. I think Nate was fine with all of this and arranged for me to get funding through an National Cancer Institute grant. During this time, I worked closely with Michael Weisman on clinical projects that included clinical trials and case series. Again, Nate was happy with all this; his laboratory was full with other trainees.

It was a time of closed community in rheumatology. I experienced that in all the places I have worked, but it was especially important in San Diego where everything was so spread out. The California motto was work to live, not live to work, and that seemed to be true of the rheumatology community. The whole region participated in a monthly conference that in those days was in person. Since clinical work was less demanding, we could look forward to conferences like these wholeheartedly, without the current anxiety about "lost productivity." Participants included colleagues from Scripps Clinic, a major referral center, Scripps Hospital, the Navy Hospital in Balboa Park, UCSD campus faculty, the San Diego Veterans Affairs Hospital, and our own rheumatology division. About 40 people generally attended. This was similar to the other city-wide rounds I had attended in Chicago, Philadelphia, and Boston. Nate always put on a good show for the luminaries from the other institutions.

Another highlight was radiology rounds with Don Resnick, an almost professional baseball player and a fellow New Rochelle High School graduate, with the world's largest collection of musculoskeletal images. Don was a showman as well. He received hard copy x-ray images from all over the world and had no hesitation showing the images and convincing us we had no clue about the disease they illustrated. Frequently, I had never heard of the disease, but most of the time Nate, Michael, and Harry knew the answer. It probably irritated Don that Nate had published the association of inflammatory bowel disease with spondylitis with Don's close colleague Bill Martel at the University of Michigan (*Arthritis and Rheumatism* 3;76–87, 1960). Conferences at UCSD were a little scary for the fellows since we needed to present at a level that challenged the attendings, hopefully not getting the dismissive "why are you presenting this?" since it was so obvious, no one would be interested. We probably should have stuck to Mexican food at the meetings since that was abundant and delicious, but Nate wanted New York–style deli, and searched high and low for pastrami on rye (that typically included mayonnaise in San Diego), usually without success.

American Rheumatology Association Meetings

We all went to the annual American Rheumatology Association (ARA) conference that rotated between various cities on the East and West coasts with an occasional Chicago thrown in for good measure. We were encouraged to submit abstracts and most of the time they were accepted for poster or podium presentation. The meetings were smaller then, probably about 5000 participants rather than the current 15,000. Nate was always surrounded by fellows and colleagues and was always generous about introducing his trainees to famous people from all over the world. He took pride in his division and the status it enjoyed as one of the elite programs. Along the way I met many of the luminaries of rheumatology, often as a direct consequence of Nate introducing me. For example, he had John Decker and Eric Bywaters as visiting scholars at UCSD. I believe he introduced me to Charles Christian from special surgery who absolutely amazed me that he remembered my name whenever we met at the ARA meetings. Sometimes Nate would find something interesting about a patient and ask us to call some expert that might have an insight. That way I got to meet Edmund DuBois and Naomi Rothfield, as well as a host of well-known rheumatologists from England and the Continent, all of whom were on a first-name basis with Nate.

The San Diego Veterans Affairs

The Veterans Affairs (VA) in San Diego was one of our required regular rotations, but not one I enjoyed. The vets had a more circumscribed set of problems, and although I was interested in gout and did some work in that disease later, it was a bit monotonous compared with the fascinating autoimmune diseases we saw downtown. The VA was up on UCSD La Jolla campus, and although there were shuttles, they were infrequent and inconvenient, so as a general rule it was a 15-mile drive up the highway, which made me feel far away from the center of my world. I never saw Nate at the VA, but our clinic there was staffed by Michael Becker who was very helpful, especially with metabolic disorders. He was followed by Bob Terkeltaub, who was to become a world leader in crystal disease.

Zvaifler's Sabbatical

Before I left San Diego, Nate went to Rockefeller to do a sabbatical in Ralph Steinman's laboratory studying dendritic cells. I had never heard of these, and neither had most rheumatologists. But as always, Nate was far ahead of everyone else in realizing the critical role these cells have in processing and presenting foreign antigens. After my fellowship, I went off to Dana Farber to study purine metabolism in more depth. Linda Thompson in Jay's laboratory introduced me to Lorraine Gudas, a postdoc at the University of California, San Francisco in David Martin's laboratory, who also studied the purinogenic immunodeficiency syndromes. Lorraine moved to Dana Farber, and I went to work in her laboratory. She left Harvard for Cornell and headed the pharmacology department there for decades. Later I was reunited with Michael Becker, another purine metabolism aficionado, who had moved to the University of Chicago to run their rheumatology division. This was a happy circumstance since the University of Chicago was a terrific place to do research and still is. There I inherited Dan McCarty's refrigerator, but sadly not his talent.

Nathan Zvaifler Chair of Medicine

Nate returned to UCSD as the interim Chairman of Medicine. This role might not have been the best fit for him because although he was the best clinician scientist at UCSD, he was not politically motivated, and frequently spoke his mind in ways that could offend thinner skinned colleagues. As it happened, a close colleague of Nate's, Steven Wasserman, an allergist/immunologist with whom I also had a 6-month clinic rotation, became the Chairman of Medicine at UCSD; Steve was much more politically adept and was very successful in this role. After I left, Harry Bluestein became the third year medical student clerkship director, and Michael Weisman went to Cedars Sinai in Los Angeles, his childhood home. Michael Weisman had a tremendous career there and recently took his prodigious skills to Stanford, where he continues to teach and mentor.

Nathan Zvaifler's History in Rheumatology

Nate grew up in New Jersey with a physician father. It was a strict upbringing. His younger brother Andrew also became a physician with a distinguished career as a physician-scientist studying hypertension at the University of Michigan. Nate went to Haverford College and graduated from Jefferson Medical College in 1952 where he was also an intern. He served as a Captain in the Air Force in Texas, returned to medical training at the University of Michigan where he was a resident, and then a fellow in the Rackham Arthritis Research Unit. He subsequently went to the National Institutes of Health for further training and then the Georgetown University School of Medicine as a faculty member. He was recruited to UCSD by Eugene Braunwald to start a rheumatology division in 1970, which he chaired for 20 years. His seminal research contribution on the immunopathogenesis of rheumatoid arthritis was published in *Advances in Immunology* 1973;16:265 to 336. He made other important contributions on the role of T cells in the rheumatoid synovium and the role of fibroblast like synoviocytes in the erosive destructive changes in the rheumatoid joint. He also contributed to the early recognition of the role of cytokines and was a close colleague of Tiny Maini, the codiscoverer of the first successfully launched tumor necrosis factor-alpha inhibitor, infliximab. He served on numerous editorial boards and was editor in chief of the journal *Arthritis and Rheumatism*, which is now *Arthritis and Rheumatology*. He received numerous awards, including Master of the American College of Rheumatology in 1993, and its gold medal in 1999.

Nathan Zvaifler's Contributions to the Field of Rheumatology

Nate's greatest contributions were those as a critical thinker, educator, and mentor to literally dozens of trainees, who uniformly came away from their exposure amazed by his brilliance, both as an astute clinician and most especially his breadth and depth of knowledge in all things rheumatologic—historical, clinical, and scientific. He taught us that it is important to learn all of rheumatology and not be pigeon holed as a lupus doctor, vasculitis doctor, or so, but to embrace all of it, and see the underlying similarities and differences in our diseases. One of his great rejoinders, when asked if we should have a lupus clinic was "If we knew who had lupus, we wouldn't need a lupus clinic." Many of his trainees, who are now toward the end of their careers, have led rheumatology divisions and kept Nate's spirit of constant inquiry alive, never satisfied with the current level of understanding of the many processes of inflammation and immune reaction that characterize the rheumatologic disorders. All of us who were fortunate enough to know and learn from him will never be able to repay the debt we owe Nate, but in mentoring budding clinicians and scientists, we honor him and ensure his remarkable legacy continues.

ACKNOWLEDGMENTS

To all the faculty and fellows at the institutions I have been affiliated with, and especially Michael Weisman, MD, a colleague and a mentor, and Christopher Burns who contributed his recollections.

DISCLOSURE

No disclosures.

FURTHER READINGS

Xu WD, Firestein GS, Taetle R, et al. Cytokines in chronic inflammatory arthritis. II. Granulocyte-macrophage colony-stimulating factor in rheumatoid synovial effusions. J Clin Invest 1989;83(3):876–82.

Primer in Rheumatic Disease John Klippel 1997 ed. Available in hard copy from Amazon and as a free download PDF document.

Pekin TJ, Zvaifler NJ. Hemolytic complement in synovial fluid. J Clin Invest 1964; 43(7):1372–82.

1989We dong Xu, Gary S. Firestein, Raymond Taetle, Kenneth Kaushansky and Nathan J. Zvaifier Journal of Clinical Investigation 83:1989 pp876-882.

Zvaifler NJ. Breakdown products of C'3 in human synovial fluid. J Clin Invest 1969;48: 1532–42.

Zvaifler J, Martel W. Spondylitis in chronic ulcerative colitis N. Arthritis Rheumatol 1960;3:pp76–87.

Zvaifler NJ. The immunopathology of joint inflammation in rheumatoid arthritis. Adv Immunol 1973;16:pp265–316.

Zvaifler J. The Immunopathology of Joint Inflammation in Rheumatoid Arthritis. Adv Immunol 1973. https://doi.org/10.1016/s0065-2776(08)60299-0.

Daniel J McCarty, MD: A Giant of Rheumatology

Ann K. Rosenthal, MD[a],*, Mary E. Csuka, MD[b],
Paul Halverson, MD[b]

KEYWORDS

- Rheumatology • Crystal arthritis • Rheumatoid arthritis
- Milwaukee shoulder syndrome • Calcium pyrophosphate deposition • Gout
- Remitting seronegative symmetric synovitis with pitting edema

KEY POINTS

- Dr Daniel J McCarty is responsible for seminal advancements in crystal arthritis in the twentieth century, including use of polarizing light microscopy and characterization of calcium pyrophosphate deposition disease and Milwaukee shoulder syndrome.
- He also contributed to major discoveries in other diseases including remitting seronegative symmetric synovitis with pitting edema (RS3PE) and triple therapy for rheumatoid arthritis.
- He was a prolific writer and international figure and as such, had major influences on the science and practice of rheumatology over the last 60 years.

INTRODUCTION

There is no doubt that Dr Daniel J McCarty (**Fig. 1**) warrants inclusion among the giants of rheumatology. He has made major contributions to both clinical and scientific knowledge in our field, and his impact has been long-lasting and paradigm shifting. He is perhaps best known for his pioneering work in crystal arthritis, but as an astute clinician, he is also responsible for describing several other novel rheumatic conditions and developing innovative treatment protocols. He successfully grew and led the academic rheumatology divisions in Chicago and Milwaukee and was the Department Chair of Medicine at the Medical College of Wisconsin (MCW). As such he has been an important mentor for many generations of physicians and scientists. Through his prolific authorship and national and international speaker engagements, his influence on rheumatology has truly been worldwide. The three of us responsible for writing this article

[a] Rheumatology Division, Medical College of Wisconsin, 6th Floor HUB Building, 9200 West Wisconsin Avenue, Milwaukee, WI 53226, USA; [b] Division of Rheumatology, Department of Medicine, Rheumatology Division, Medical College of Wisconsin, 6th Floor HUB Building, 9200 West Wisconsin Avenue, Milwaukee, WI 53226, USA
* Corresponding author.
E-mail address: arosenthal@mcw.edu

Rheum Dis Clin N Am 50 (2024) 15–23
https://doi.org/10.1016/j.rdc.2023.08.001
0889-857X/24/© 2023 Elsevier Inc. All rights reserved.

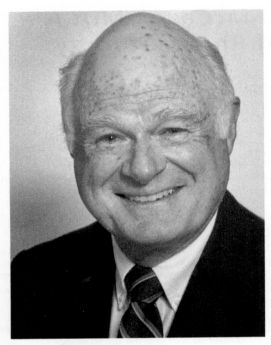

Fig. 1. Photograph of Dr Daniel J McCarty.

have had the privilege of working with Dr McCarty at MCW for many years. As he is alive and well at the time we are writing this, we welcomed his input and have included some personal anecdotes and remembrances scattered throughout this article.

EDUCATION AND POSITIONS

Dr McCarty was born in Philadelphia in 1928. He attended college at Villanova University and medical school at the University of Pennsylvania School of Medicine, where he was elected to the Alpha Omega Alpha Honor Society. After his graduation in 1954 and a year of internship, he volunteered for military service. He spent the years 1957 to 1959 in the army and was stationed in Germany where he ran a dispensary. On returning to the United States, he recalls being somewhat uncertain as to a choice of specialty but commenced training as a dermatology resident. In his own words, the length of training, lack of satisfaction with the area (and low pay) caused him to look elsewhere. He considered pursuing hematology, but training was not available locally. He approached Dr Joseph Hollander about a position. At the time, Dr Hollander was a major figure in rheumatology and was editor of the premiere textbook in the field. Dr Hollander was able to obtain National Institute of Health (NIH) funding for Dr McCarty for 1 year of training which included doing rheumatology research and his experience during this critical year firmly established his ultimate career direction. Dr McCarty joined the faculty as an assistant professor at the University of Pennsylvania School of Medicine in 1960. After 3 years there, he left for Hahnemann Medical College where he was promoted to an associate professor in 1963. He then left Philadelphia in 1967 to join the faculty of the University of Chicago School of Medicine as a full professor and the Head of the Section of Arthritis and Metabolic Disease. He spent 1971 in

Bern, Switzerland, as a visiting professor. In 1974, he relocated to Milwaukee, WI, and joined the faculty at MCW as the Chairman of the Department of Medicine. In 1989, he became the Will and Cava Ross Professor of Medicine. At MCW, he built an impressive rheumatology division and a strong department of medicine. He remained at MCW until his retirement in 2000. His career is certainly notable in many ways, but his meteoric rise through the academic ranks and his appointment as a department chair at age 47 years clearly suggest an early recognition of his many talents.

CHOICE OF A RESEARCH FIELD AND MENTOR

When Dr Hollander offered Dr McCarty a year of funded research at the University of Pennsylvania in 1960, rheumatology was just developing. Dr McCarty recalls a scene in which Dr Hollander set up a microscope with a slide of joint fluid from a patient believed to have gout. The dark structures in the microscope field were not distinctive. When asked by Dr Hollander what the crystals were, Dr McCarty replied, "I don't know," because the identity of urate had not been proven using microscopy. Dr Hollander was a little surprised at his response. Subsequently, Dr Hollander left Philadelphia to spend the summer in Maine and assigned Dr McCarty the task of finding a means of confirming the identity of urate crystals. At the University of Pennsylvania, there was a Department of Crystallography, but crystals in joint fluid were not easily amenable to standard crystallographic techniques. He was advised to ask for help from the Department of Botany because they had a polarizing light microscope. Thus, each time he wanted to examine joint fluids, this required a two-block walk to the facility that housed the polarizing microscope. The first specimen he examined contained scrapings from a gouty tophus. He recalls that the sight under polarized light microscopy of this mass of negatively birefringent crystals was quite beautiful (**Fig. 2**) . Subsequently, he collected synovial fluids from patients and began to examine them. To his surprise, several fluids demonstrated weakly positively birefringent crystals (**Fig. 3**) in contrast to the needle-shaped negatively birefringent gout crystals. His first thought was that this technique was not going to be useful to conclusively prove the presence of urate crystals. However, within a few weeks of examining clinical specimens, he became convinced that there were two different types of

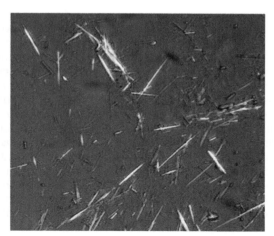

Fig. 2. Urate crystals. Urate crystals appear as brightly birefringent needle-shaped crystals under polarizing light microscopy.

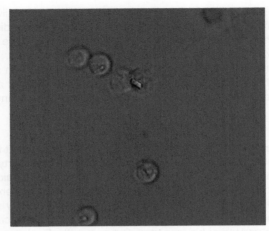

Fig. 3. Calcium pyrophosphate crystals. Calcium pyrophosphate crystals appear as rhomboidal crystals in cells under polarizing light microscopy.

crystals. His first paper presented to the American Rheumatism Association was not in a plenary session, but this new information was very well received. Dr Hollander gave his blessing to Dr McCarty to pursue research on crystal arthritis and thus began his amazingly productive career.

PERSONAL LIFE/ATTRIBUTES

Dr McCarty's immediate family grew exponentially during his early career. He married his childhood sweetheart, Constance Paakh, in 1954, the year he graduated from medical school, and they had five children between 1956 and 1966. He is now the proud grandfather of nine grandchildren and one great grandchild. After retirement, he made a clean break with science and medicine to spend time with his wife, children, and grandchildren. He enjoyed writing poetry and worked on a history of medicine. He is the author of several published poems. One of our particular favorites is "Ode to Articular Cartilage."[1] This work highlights his gregarious polymath persona and clear charm. Outside of work, he is widely known for his unique sense of humor and his interesting observations about people and society. While at work, he made his high expectations, attention to detail, and serious work ethic known to all. These standards even applied to the dress code, and we recall him sending home medical residents who were not wearing appropriate neckwear! As evidenced below, he was a master of clinical observation. He had an uncanny ability to recognize unique patterns in patients, which resulted in the description of several important clinical syndromes. He was also a very brave clinician. He dealt with the uncertainty that is intrinsic in our field with considerable confidence. For example, his early use of triple therapy in rheumatoid arthritis (RA) required quite an adventurous spirit. He was also an extremely brave scientist. When he injected himself (and a dog) with gout crystals to prove Koch's postulates, he (and the dog) experienced extreme pain for the sake of science.[2] Obviously, this occurred before the current level of human research oversight provided by institutional review boards, but this work was published and received with considerable acclaim.

ACADEMIC CONTRIBUTIONS

Dr McCarty made many contributions locally, nationally, and internationally to the field through his extensive published works. He was a prolific editor of textbooks and journals. He served as the Editor-in Chief of "Arthritis and Rheumatology" from 1965 to 1970. He was co-editor and then editor of the textbook, Arthritis and Allied Conditions, which was the premiere textbook of rheumatology at that time and was originally edited by Joseph Hollander. He was a founding editor of "Current Opinion in Rheumatology." He served on the editorial board of JAMA from 1982 to 1990. He made major contributions to the American College of Physicians, the American Federation for Clinical Research, and the American College of Rheumatology (ACR), where he served as president from 1989 to 1990. He was also an active member of the highly selective society known as the American Clinical and Climatologic Association (ACCA). This is a small group of physicians from across the spectrum of medicine, who have devoted themselves to medical education, science, and climate change. Interestingly, the ACCA began in 1988 as an elite group of physicians interested in the study of tuberculosis. Of note, Dr McCarty is the author of over 300 publications, including original research and many invited chapters and reviews.

HONORS AND AWARDS

Dr McCarty has received numerous awards over his long career. Notable are the AMAs Hektoen medal awarded in 1963, the Heberden Oration and Gold medal from the Heberden Society in London, England, and the Joseph Bunim Lecturer and Gold Medal from the American Rheumatism Association (the predecessor of the ACR) in 1984. He ultimately attained Master Status at the ACR. He gave talks all over the world and was a member of many national rheumatology organizations including those in New Zealand, Indonesia, and Argentina. His curriculum vitae lists invited lectures in no less than 33 different countries. He was the first Nanna Svartz Memorial Lecturer in Stockholm, Sweden, and was named an alpha omega alpha (AOA) leader in medicine in the oral history program in 1997. In the state of Wisconsin, he was a Middleton lecturer and received the Wisconsin Laureate Award from the state chapter of the American College of Physicians in 1997. As a way to honor his work at MCW, the Department of Medicine now has a "Daniel J McCarty Award" given annually to mid-career faculty in recognition of their research achievements.

MENTORSHIP/ACADEMIC LEGACY

Dr McCarty was an amazing mentor to the three authors of this article, and in general, took great interest in supporting younger physicians and their careers. Dr Lawrence M Ryan, who is responsible for most of the exceptional work on calcium pyrophosphate (CPP) crystal formation, was the first rheumatology fellow at MCW and was a close research colleague of Dr McCarty's. This work has been continued by Dr Rosenthal. Dr McCarty also had major influences on the careers of many other rheumatologists. This list includes Geraldine McCarthy, Frank Kozin, Robert Wortmann, Ikuko Masuda, John Rachow, and many others. Dr McCarty was particularly welcoming to international students, residents, and fellows, many of whom brought back essential clinical and research skills to their native countries. Dr McCarty's legacy at MCW is certainly long-lasting. He worked diligently to raise money for endowments designed to support both educational and research-related pursuits. Many grateful patients gave money to the institution because of his excellent clinical care and his impressive research accomplishments. These funds have supported numerous enterprising faculty members in the department of medicine and the rheumatology division at MCW.

CONTRIBUTIONS TO RHEUMATOLOGY

The use of polarized light microscopy for crystal arthritis: As noted above, Dr McCarty's early contributions related to the use of polarizing microscopy for diagnosing crystal arthritis. His first paper on his topic was published with Joseph Hollander in 1961.[3] They described the typical morphology and birefringent characteristics of monosodium urate (MSU) crystals in synovial fluid and proved that they dissolved with uricase exposure. They proposed the use of this technology as a highly reliable diagnostic test for gout. The impact of this work in the crystal field was major and two-pronged. Before the application of polarized light microscopy to synovial fluid analysis, the diagnosis of gout was based on serum urate levels or classic x-ray changes. We know now that reliance on these features often leads to inaccurate diagnoses. Even more importantly, however, some of the fluids originally examined in this paper contained crystals that were not composed of urate. A sentence in the discussion of the paper states, "The finding of definitely non-urate crystals in the joint fluid from an otherwise typical case of acute gouty arthritis even suggests the possibility of a hitherto unrecognized metabolic abnormality which can mimic the syndrome of gout."[3] Thus, calcium pyrophosphate deposition disease (CPPD) was born.

Calcium pyrophosphate deposition disease identification, clinical characterization and pathogenesis: As one not apt to leave such an interesting observation unexplored, Dr McCarty set out to determine the nature of these uricase-resistant synovial fluid crystals. He rapidly discovered that these crystals were composed of calcium PPi dihydrate, and very soon,[4] he published the first descriptions of the now commonly recognized arthritis initially known as pseudogout and now called CPPD. Dr McCarty devoted much of his research time in the early years after this discovery describing and carefully documenting the clinical presentations and disease course of patients with this type of crystal deposition. He noted the high prevalence in the elderly as well as discovered kindreds with early-onset severe familial disease. He made the connections with the co-morbid conditions known to be associated with CPPD including hypophosphatasia, hyperparathyroidism, hypomagnesemia, and hemochromatosis. His diagnostic criteria and etiologic classification scheme for CPPD remain the only published work of its kind to date.

Because he was not one to focus solely on the clinical aspects of a disease, once he was comfortably ensconced as the department chair at MCW, Dr McCarty set out to explore the pathophysiology of CPPD. He built a group of physician investigators, PhD scientists, and talented laboratory personnel to address issues of causation. Incredible minds such as Lawrence M Ryan, John Rachow, Robert Wortmann, and many talented rheumatology fellows and others set out to determine how CPPD crystals are formed. Dr McCarty recruited Herman Cheung, PhD, to start his own laboratory focused on crystal arthritis and had visiting scientists from Ireland, Japan, and Korea working on these projects. During the early years at MCW and based on some work from the Seegmiller laboratory,[5] the group worked diligently to measure PPi, the anionic component of CPP crystals. This was a difficult task, and the radiometric assay that they constructed is still today the most accurate and sensitive assay in use. Dr Ryan showed that PPi was present in synovial fluid in concentrations higher in patients with CPPD than non-crystal controls and delineated the mechanisms through which PPi was made by chondrocytes and the factors that affected calcium PPi crystal formation. This work has been essential to the field, and MCW remains one of the few sites in the world actively doing research devoted to uncovering the secrets of CPPD crystal formation.

Milwaukee Shoulder and basic calcium phosphate crystals: In the mid-1970s, several elderly women came to Dr McCarty's clinic with severe shoulder damage. The main features were pain, limited motion, sometimes massive shoulder effusions (hydrops), and bland synovial fluids lacking evidence of inflammation. Some of these patients had CPPD crystals, large rotator cuff tears, and humeral head remodeling which were not typical of simple osteoarthritic changes. His laboratory was able to assess the joint fluids which had been aspirated for the presence of basic calcium phosphate (BCP) crystals using a radiometric assay and electron microscopy. Interestingly, fluids demonstrated the presence of collagenase which was hypothesized to be responsible for the widespread tissue destruction in these patients. This condition was described as Milwaukee shoulder syndrome, but also described in the orthopedic literature as "cuff tear arthropathy." The exact relationship of BCP crystals to arthritis has not been clearly elucidated. In vitro studies showed that BCP crystals stimulated the production of collagenase and prostaglandins in cultures of synovial fibroblasts. Studies such as these suggested that BCP crystals might amplify an ongoing pathogenic process such as osteoarthritis. Much of this work published in the last 20 years has been from Dr Geraldine McCarthy, who started her career with Dr McCarty.

RS3PE: This interesting condition was described in 1985 in a case collection of patients with seronegative inflammatory arthritis published by Drs. McCarty, Desmond O'Duffy, Larry Pearson, and Jay B Hunter in JAMA.[6] They described eight men and two women with inflammatory arthritis of subacute onset affecting large and small joints and characterized by pitting edema in the hands and feet. This dramatic type of arthritis typically affected individuals more than the age of 60 years and had an excellent response to aspirin and hydroxychloroquine. It represented a clinical overlap between polymyalgia rheumatica and seronegative RA yet remains today a clearly distinct clinical syndrome. In the ensuing 38 years since its description, this intriguing syndrome has received increasing attention as a possible paraneoplastic process and may result from inflammatory pathways involving interleukin (IL)-6 and vascular endothelial growth factor (VEGF).[7]

Triple therapy for rheumatoid arthritis: Dr McCarty was a dedicated clinician frustrated by the limited effectiveness of available drug treatments for RA, with hydroxychloroquine, gold, and/or penicillamine being the only FDA-approved drug therapies. During the 1960s and 1970s, the observation that the thiopurine, azathioprine, provided benefit in RA suggested the efficacy of immunosuppressive therapy, but never received FDA approval. Drug toxicity was considered of more concern than the deleterious effects of uncontrolled inflammation. Furthermore, treatment starts were often delayed until the first erosion was identified and then discontinued once remission achieved only to have disease activity return. This paradigm has been replaced with recommendations to begin drug treatment at the time of diagnosis and not to discontinue treatment once control of the inflammatory process was achieved.

Dr Mc Carty was an early pioneer in the concept of using combination drug therapy for RA, a concept he borrowed from the treatment of hematologic malignancies. To set the stage in 1982, in the background of his first paper on the subject, he described the current state of the art for managing RA, "as establishment of a good basic program (avoidance of severe physical demands on the affected joints, range of motion exercises, supportive shoes) coupled with gold compounds, aspirin or other cyclooxygenase inhibitors, intra-articular corticosteroid injections and perhaps 5 to 10 mg of prednisone."[8] In this paper, he described 17 patients with intractable RA, who he treated with the combination of low-dose cyclophosphamide, azathioprine, and hydroxychloroquine. Disease suppression was achieved in 14/17 and complete remission in 5/17. He noted the experimental nature of the regimen and recommended its use for a select group of highly refractory patients. This work introduced and gave credence to the concept of using smaller doses of multiple potent drugs in combination to approach this disease. Unfortunately, in a follow-up study published in 1986,[9] he concluded that although this approach had promise, a high rate of malignancy (12%), including one patient with erythroleukemia, warranted replacement of the cyclophosphamide with a non-alkylating agent. This important concept of adding a second or third drug rather than continued monotherapy was developed further and is still in use today with a different set of RA drugs.[10]

SUMMARY

Dr McCarty is a true giant of rheumatology. His clinical and scientific discoveries made a major impact on our specialty, and many patients have benefited from his work. He has been an exceptional mentor and role model to many generations of physicians and was a true "triple threat" during his long and productive career. All three of the authors of this article had the great privilege to know and work with him. We can attest to the major positive impact he has had on our own clinical practice styles, the value we place on clinical observation, and the way in which we approach scientific questions. We all feel extremely lucky to have had our professional lives enriched by his presence and greatly enjoyed describing his exceptional talents and summarizing his amazing career in this article.

CLINICS CARE POINTS

- Clinical observations are critical to the advancement of medical knowledge.
- Given time, resources, and an inquiring mind, even junior physicians can make amazing contributions to a field.

DISCLOSURES

None of the authors have financial disclosures related to this work. Some of the material is the result of work supported with resources and the use of facilities at the Zablocki VA Medical Center in Milwaukee, WI. The contents do not represent the views of the US Department of Veterans Affairs or the United States Government.

REFERENCES

1. McCarty DJ. That Ode Feeling. Arthritis Rheum 1981;24:1455.
2. Faires J, McCarty D Jr. Acute arthritis in man and dog after intrasynovial injection of sodium urate crystals. Lancet 1962;280(7258):682–5.
3. McCarty DJ, Hollander JL. Identification of urate crystals in gouty synovial fluid. Ann Intern Med 1961;54:452–60.
4. McCarty D, Kohn N, Faires J. The significance of calcium pyrophosphate crystals in the synovial fluid of arthritic patients. 1. Clinical aspects. Ann Intern Med 1962; 56:711–37.

5. Lust G, Faure G, Netter P, et al. Increased pyrophosphate in fibroblasts and lymphoblasts from patients with hereditary diffuse articular chondrocalcinosis. Science 1981;214(4522):809–10.
6. McCarty DJ, O'Duffy JD, Pearson L, et al. Remitting seronegative symmetrical synovitis with pitting edema. RS3PE syndrome. Jama. 1985;254(19):2763–7.
7. Borges T, Silva S. RS3PE Syndrome: Autoinflammatory Features of a Rare Disorder. Mod Rheumatol 2022. https://doi.org/10.1093/mr/roac071.
8. McCarty DJ, Carrera GF. Intractable rheumatoid arthritis. Treatment with combined cyclophosphamide, azathioprine, and hydroxychloroquine. JAMA 1982; 248(14):1718–23.
9. Csuka M, Carrera GF, McCarty DJ. Treatment of intractable rheumatoid arthritis with combined cyclophosphamide, azathioprine, and hydroxychloroquine. A follow-up study. JAMA 1986;255(17):2315–9.
10. O'Dell JR. Triple therapy with methotrexate, sulfasalazine, and hydroxychloroquine in patients with rheumatoid arthritis. Rheum Dis Clin N Am 1998;24(3):465–77.

Gerald P Rodnan

Virginia D. Steen, MD[a],*, Thomas A. Medsger, MD[b]

KEYWORDS

- Systemic sclerosis • Rheumatology • Modified Rodnan skin score • Uric acid

KEY POINTS

- Dr Rodnan's passion for scleroderma, gout, history of medicine and education stimulated many to have this 'infectious' passion as well.
- The clinical and pathologic studies that he did scleroderma led to a better overall understanding of the disease.
- The modified Rodnan Skin Score, originated by Dr. Rodnan remains the gold standard for evaluating extent and severity of skin thickening in scleroderma.

Gerald P Rodnan, MD, was a true savant (**Fig. 1**). He was very knowledgeable in multiple scientific areas, including systemic sclerosis (SSc) (scleroderma), gout, and the history of medicine. He had an intense interest in all of these topics which resulted in numerous significant contributions to the medical literature. In addition, he was passionate about teaching and patient care and superb as a bedside teacher and lecturer. Both of us served as rheumatology fellows and full-time faculty members under Gerry, who greatly influenced our careers in academic medicine by steering us to focus on SSc.

EDUCATION, TRAINING, AND FAMILY

Dr Rodnan graduated from Long Island College of Medicine (now State University of New York) in 1949. He did an internship at Maimonides Hospital in New York before going to Duke University to complete his internal medicine residency. He next was invited to be a Clinical Investigator at the National Institutes of Health under the supervision of the late Dr Joseph Bunin, who stimulated his interest in rheumatology. Gerry published on metabolic liver disease,[1] the metabolism of gout,[2] gout in African American females,[3] and the anemia associated with rheumatic diseases.[4] Bunin introduced him to the world of scleroderma which resulted in a report of the use of corticosteroids in SSc.[5] In 1955, Rodnan was recruited to the University of Pittsburgh School of Medicine where he became the first Chief of the Division of Rheumatology and Clinical

[a] Georgetown University School of Medicine, 3800 Reservoir Road, PHC 3004, Washington, DC 20007, USA; [b] University of Pittsburgh School of Medicine, 3550 Terrace Street, Pittsburgh, PA 15213, USA
* Corresponding author. 3800 Reservoir Road, PHC 3004, Washington, DC 20007.
E-mail address: steenv@georgetown.edu

Rheum Dis Clin N Am 50 (2024) 25–32
https://doi.org/10.1016/j.rdc.2023.08.002
0889-857X/24/© 2023 Elsevier Inc. All rights reserved.

rheumatic.theclinics.com

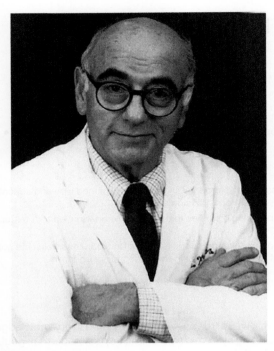

Fig. 1. Gerald P Rodnan, MD, 1980.

Immunology, a position which he held until his premature death at the age of 56 years in 1983. He was a prolific writer. Despite his unfortunately short career, he published 180 refereed articles and 22 textbook chapters. Rodnan established the Rheumatology Fellowship Program with the first 2 year graduates completing training in 1963. More than 40 fellows completed the program under his direction, including MD/PhD researchers and international scholars. Thereafter, they did research or practice in 13 states and 7 countries.

Gerry's wife Joan was a full-time faculty member at the Pitt's Department of Pediatrics and was the Director of the Cystic Fibrosis program. She died barely 1 month after Gerry. Their children, Leslie, Meredith, and Andrew went on to have careers in pediatric genetics, speech therapy, and business/real estate, respectively, and all of them settled in the Washington DC area.

PERSONAL CHARACTERISTICS AND HABITS

At conferences and meetings, Gerry was witty and incisive in his analysis of cases and the medical literature. In public, he could be the "life of the party," but on occasion, he seemed quiet and preoccupied. Gerry loved to eat and enjoyed cigars. A well-known silhouette caricature shows him with a fat cigar in his mouth.

He was a meticulous writer and editor. He spent many hours rewriting and perfecting manuscripts, both his own and those of colleagues and trainees. His "touch" with words made his descriptions very relatable and meaningful, more like reading a novel than a dry scientific paper. He was compulsive about using precise grammar, interpreting literature, and correctly recording references. His written and lecture illustrations (clinical, radiologic, pathologic/photomicrographic) were superb. He worked closely with an outstanding local medical illustrator to produce these excellent images.

Gerry was the editor of the Bulletin on the Rheumatic Diseases (1966–1982), a 6 to 8 page quarterly publication which he transformed into one of the most widely read educational periodicals in rheumatology. He edited the 7th and 8th editions of the Primer on the Rheumatic Diseases and had the vision to expand this to a 60 to 80 page "go to" volume with up-to-date chapters by well-recognized experts, with content primarily written for medical students, residents, and fellows.

Gerry thoroughly enjoyed traveling and serving as a guest lecturer/visiting professor. He lectured in all but one of the 48 continental states (Wyoming). He had to cancel a trip to Cheyenne because of illness and was unable to "complete the circuit" before his death. He personally knew, visited and frequently corresponded with almost all of the giants in rheumatology honored in this book. He exchanged signed head and shoulders photographs with many of these prominent men and women, which he displayed on the walls of the Fellows' Conference Room.

Gerry's unique data collection method consisted of 4 × 6 inch index cards on which he recorded an incredible amount of demographic, occupational, and clinical data. For example, he documented the date of onset of each organ system affected by scleroderma, including specifics history, physical examination, and laboratory findings. This rich data set formed the basis for the later development of the computer-based Pittsburgh Scleroderma Database, which includes first and follow-up visit data on more than 5000 SSc patients first evaluated at Pitt between 1972 and the present. Rodnan personally did one or more "punch" skin biopsies on more than 600 scleroderma patients. He was especially devoted to all of his patients with this disease and their family members. Whenever possible, he obtained and carefully studied the autopsies of deceased SSc patients and routinely attended patients' funerals.

NATIONAL AND INTERNATIONAL ACTIVITIES

Gerry was active in the American Rheumatism Association (ARA), which was then part of the Arthritis Foundation, predating the American College of Rheumatology (ACR). He helped to organize an interim meeting of the ARA which was held in Pittsburgh in 1973 and attracted 750 participants with a bargain registration fee of $10! Dr Rodnan was elected the President of the ARA for 1975 to 1976. Not surprisingly, his 1976 presidential address focused on changes in rheumatology over the preceding two centuries. In 1776, there were only two recognized rheumatic diseases, gout and "arthritis," the number of which grew to nearly 100 distinct conditions by 1976. By this 40th ARA annual meeting, he noted that there were 2500 ARA members, yet at the same time 26 states had fewer than 10 trained rheumatologists.[6]

Gerry was recognized worldwide as the "father of scleroderma." His lectures were akin to sermons in which he animatedly "preached" the need for all physicians to recognize the manifestations of this disease and its variants and to make this diagnosis with confidence. Interestingly, his favorite "sclerodermatologist" was not a rheumatologist, but rather a highly respected and productive academic dermatologist, Professor Stephania Jablonska, Director of the Scleroderma Clinic in the Department of Dermatology at the University of Warsaw in Poland. They saw each other often at scientific meetings and frequently exchanged letters, both about their scleroderma activities and a wide variety of other mutual interests.

GOUT, ALCOHOL, AND PURINE INTAKE

Dr Rodnan was fascinated by the metabolism of uric acid and the physiology of its excretion, which led to a research publication in the Journal of Clinical Investigation.[2] He was aware of the numerous published cartoons which called attention to the occurrence of gout in English aldermen (public officials) and their associated obesity, excessive intake of meat and alcohol, typically Port wine. Rodnan introduced the term "aldermanic gout" to describe this concurrence.[7] To study the entity more specifically, he admitted known gout sufferers to our Clinical Research Unit and fed them a high-purine diet and followed their hourly serum uric acid levels and urinary excretion of beta-hydroxybutyrate and acetoacetate, both of which were considered to reduce urinary uric acid excretion and thus increase serum levels of uric acid (SUA). After a 1-day "recovery," the high-purine diet was given again, this time with the addition of one ounce of alcohol per hour from 4:00 PM until midnight. The result was a rapid increase in serum uric acid, up by an average of 3 mg/dL with meat and as much as 6 mg/dL when alcohol was added. As expected, in some cases, acute gouty arthritis occurred at or shortly after peak SUA was reached.[8,9] As fellows responsible for these research unit patients, both of us had to deal with the acute gout episodes as well as sometimes unruly behavior which followed such "forced" high alcohol intake. Rodnan was the first to demonstrate that the xanthine oxidase inhibitor allopurinol does not require multiple daily doses and is equally effective when given as a single daily dose.[10]

Rodnan's true love was the history of gout. Early in his career, he published "A Gallery of Gout" in Arthritis and Rheumatism.[11] He and his long-time friend and colleague, Dr Thomas G Benedek, Chief of Rheumatology at the Pittsburgh Veterans Administration Hospital, wrote numerous articles and coauthored several books on the history of medicine and gout. Rodnan was a voracious collector of rare books on these subjects. His entire collection of more than 650 volumes was donated to the University of Pittsburgh's Falk Medical Library by his children in 1985, at which time the room in which his and other books of historical significance are housed was renamed the Rodnan Rare Book Room. Some of the holdings include several sixteenth-century gout treatises by Pirckheimer (in German), Gout's Apology (1522),[12] and Gout Manual by Ferro in Spanish (1584).[13]

We participated in a classic Rodnan history of gout book anecdote. In 1982, while intubated in the Intensive Care Unit, his secretary brought him his daily mail, which often included rare book catalogs. After perusing one, he wrote her a terse note on a pad as follows: "Buy this book. $2000. Checkbook in office desk top drawer." She dutifully found the check book, then panicked when she saw that he had a joint checking account with his wife. She asked one of us (TAM) what to do. Given the circumstance and his insistence, I told her to write the check for his signature and purchase the book. Two months later, although he was recovering at home, the book arrived at the academic office. It was an original 1683 Latin edition of Thomas Sydenham's Tractatus de Podagra et Hydrope…(Tract on Gout and Dropsy).[14] Although he already had several English editions, this Latin edition was truly rare. The other of us (VDS) had the pleasure of delivering the book to Rodnan at his home. He was incredibly happy, profusely thanked me and commented "This is the best day of my life!" As it turned out, the book is the Rare Book Room's most celebrated volume and had an estimated value of over $4000!

Rodnan voraciously collected original gout prints from book stores all over the world. He amassed more than 400 prints which are currently housed in Washington DC. In 1984, his children generously gave the Rheumatology Research Foundation permission to reproduce a limited number of copies of selected prints for sale as a fundraiser at each annual ACR meeting which they did for 25 years.

Colleagues have complained that Rodnan was highly competitive, "beating out" rival collectors for prints, as Eric Bywaters noted concerning an antiquities bookstore in London.[15] John Baum, a pediatric rheumatologist from Rochester, NY, and friend of Rodnan, recalled getting interested in gout prints and visiting a book store (librairie) in

Paris and inquiring about prints. The proprietor said "I don't have any. When I get one, I sell it to a fat man from Pittsburgh."

Rodnan himself suffered all of the manifestations of "metabolic syndrome," including occasional episodes of gouty arthritis. During one podagra attack, he insisted that one of us (TAM) go to the hospital, get a vial of colchicine for intravenous use and inject him, whereas he sat in his office with a red, hot swollen foot elevated on a classic gout stool. Our feeling was that somewhat perversely he considered it a privilege to have gout attacks and clearly wanted to experience the significant and rapid relief so often felt after administration of intravenous colchicine.

SYSTEMIC SCLEROSIS (SCLERODERMA)

Gerry's first Pittsburgh SSc patient publication was a logical continuation of his National Institutes of Health (NIH) interest in the effects of corticosteroids on the natural history of the disease. Here, he raised the caution that the use of high-dose steroids may precipitate scleroderma renal crisis (SRC),[16] an observation later confirmed in a large study by his Pittsburgh group.[17] Rodnan rapidly accumulated a sizable cohort of SSc patients in the western PA region. He established working research relationships with specialists in pulmonary medicine, cardiology, gastroenterology, and nephrology as well as radiology and pathology, to facilitate a comprehensive approach to patient care, research, and teaching. He published his observations on the first 300 Pittsburgh SSc patients in 1963.[18] Such collaborations resulted in several subsequent articles on distinctive features of the disease, including joint involvement and palpable tendon friction rubs,[19] low diffusing capacity of carbon monoxide as an early pulmonary disease sign,[20] pulmonary arterial hypertension,[21] and identification of the variant without cutaneous involvement, SSc sine scleroderma.[22] He also had several very important papers with pathologists on renal, lung, vasculature, and skin involvement,[16,20,23,24] and particularly, he very carefully characterized the histochemical, immunologic, and electron microscopy findings of scleroderma blood vessels and skin.[23,24] He was one of the first to report successful use of captopril to reverse SRC.[25]

Gerry looked for "kindred spirits" across the country to stimulate interest in the study of SSc who included several of this book's Giants (E Carwile LeRoy, Naomi Rothfield, Larry Shulman) and other researchers. These individuals met informally at annual ACR meetings. When it became clear that SSc patients frequently had positive serum antinuclear antibody tests, often with speckled nuclear staining.[26] Gerry named the group the "Speckled Band." Such groups were a precursor of rheumatic disease-related study groups which became popular in rheumatology during subsequent decades and continue today, some with hundreds of members and numerous group-sponsored collaborative research projects. With funding from the RGK Foundation, Rodnan organized an international 4-day International Conference on Progressive Systemic Sclerosis in Austin, TX, in 1981, which attracted 150 participants. Abstracts of the proceedings were published posthumously in 1985.[27]

An important feature of the Pittsburgh Scleroderma Database was the routine collection and storage of serum at the first evaluation. This innovation ultimately resulted in important observations on the clinical associations of multiple new SSc-specific serum autoantibodies and the development of the now widely accepted concept of the clinical-serologic classification of SSc.[28,29]

The most enduring Rodnan contribution to SSc was the creation of a semiquantitative bedside method for grading skin thickening, particularly useful in the diffuse cutaneous form of the disease.[30] This system was based on a 0 to 4 grading of skin thickness at 26 cutaneous anatomic sites on physical examination (**Fig. 2**). Addition

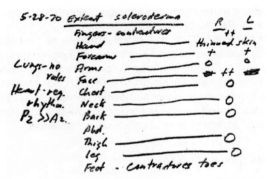

Fig. 2. Dr Rodnan patient record from 1970 illustrating a precursor of the Rodnan skin thickness scoring method first published in 1979.

of scores at each of these sites yields a total skin thickness score (maximum 104). Rodnan showed that skin scores from the forearm were strongly correlated with the dry weight of skin punch biopsies from the same location.[31] The original method was modified later to a 0 to 3 grading of 17 cutaneous sites (modified Rodnan skin score [mRSS]; maximum 51).[32,33] The mRSS remains the gold standard for measurement of skin thickness in diffuse SSc clinical trials, where it is most often the primary endpoint, and in observational studies.

GERRY RODNAN AND LARRY SHULMAN

Gerry and Larry Shulman (Johns Hopkins) were good friends yet fierce rivals. When the textbook Arthritis and Related Diseases was the rheumatologist's bible, its editors, such as Dan McCarty, had great difficulty in convincing Rodnan and Shulman to submit their chapters on SSc and lupus, respectively, in a timely manner. Why? The answer was simple—delaying allowed a chapter to be the most current with up-to-date references. Neither Gerry nor Larry wanted to submit his chapter until receiving confirmation that the other had done so, thus infuriating the editor.

In January, 1974, at the Toronto Interim Meeting of the ARA, I (TAM) heard Shulman describe four patients with the scleroderma mimic "diffuse fasciitis with eosinophilia" (DFE).[34] I immediately knew that the Pittsburgh Database included several of these cases which we had not recognized. Gerry, who had not attended the Toronto meeting, was unconvinced when he read the abstract. I told him I planned to send one of our patients to Shulman for confirmation. The latter was delighted to confirm DFE and to imply that Rodnan had missed the correct diagnosis. Rodnan, of course, was infuriated by my audacious referral and the subsequent teasing by Shulman. But perhaps Rodnan had the last laugh. Over the next several years, he scoured our database and looked carefully at all new patients, eventually identifying 20 patients with the typical clinical and fascial pathologic features of DFE, published them and suggested the name "eosinophilic fasciitis", a term which supplanted DFE in common clinical usage.[35]

SUMMARY

Dr Gerald Rodnan was a man of many talents who developed a single-minded fascination with the disease SSc. His passion and vision led to numerous important research contributions to our understanding of the natural history of this disease and his extensive travel and teaching stimulated many other investigators in the United States and throughout the world to devote their careers to this uncommon but serious disorder. He indeed was a "Giant" in rheumatology and those of us who had the opportunity to train under him have been inspired to carry it forward.

CLINICS CARE POINTS

- Xanthine oxidase inhibitors can be used as a single daily dose.
- Tendon friction rubs are a helpful sign of diffuse cutaneous scleroderma.
- Pulmonary arterial hypertension is a deadly complication in scleroderma, particularly in CREST syndrome, known now as limited cutaneous scleroderma.
- Eosinophilic fasciitis is a distinct entity which is a mimic of systemic sclerosis.

DISCLOSURE

The authors have no disclosures related to this publication.

REFERENCES

1. Chernick SS, Moe JG, Rodnan GP, et al. A metabolic lesion in dietary necrotic liver degeneration. J Biol Chem 1955;21:829–43.
2. Lathem W, Rodnan GP. Impairment of uric acid excretion in gout. J Clin Invest 1962;41:1955–63.
3. Rodnan GP, Golomb MW. Gout in the Negro female. Am J Med Sci 1958;236: 269–83.
4. Ebaugh FG Jr, Peterson RE, Rodnan GP, et al. The anemia of rheumatoid arthritis. Med Clin North Am 1955;12:489–98.
5. Rodnan GP, Black RL, Bollet AJ, et al. Observations on the use of prednisone in patients with progressive systemic sclerosis (diffuse scleroderma). Ann Intern Med 1956;44:16–29.
6. Rodnan GP. Growth and development of rheumatology in the United States–a bicentennial report. Presidential address to the American Rheumatism Association. Arthritis Rheum 1977;20:1149–68.
7. Kedar E, Simkin PA. A perspective on diet and gout. Adv Chronic Kidney Dis 2012;19:392–7.
8. Rodnan GP. The pathogenesis of aldermanic gout: procatarctic role of fluctuations in serum urate concentration in gouty arthritis provoked by feast and alcohol [abstract]. Arthritis Rheum 1980;23(suppl):737.
9. Rodnan GP. Early theories concerning etiology and pathogenesis of the gout. Arthritis Rheum 1965;8:599–610.
10. Rodnan GP, Robin JA, Tolchin SF. Efficacy of single daily dose allopurinol in gouty hyperuricemia. Adv Exp Med Biol 1974;41:571–5.
11. Rodnan GP. A gallery of gout. Being a miscellany of prints and caricatures from the 16th century to the present day. Arthritis Rheum 1961;4:27–46.
12. Pirckheimer W. Apologia seu Podagrae laus (German) published Nuremberg, 1522. HSLS Update; 2013.
13. Ferri DA. De podagra enchiridion (Latin) published Naples, 1584.
14. Sydenham T. Tractatus de podagra et hydrope (Tract on gout and dropsy) (Latin), Published England, 1683.

15. Bywaters EGL. Obituary: Gerald P Rodnan. Br J Rheumatol 1984;3:152–3.
16. Rodnan GP, Schreiner GE, Black RL. Renal involvement in progressive systemic sclerosis (generalized scleroderma). Am J Med 1957;23:445–62.
17. Steen VD. Medsger TA Case-control study of corticosteroids and other drugs that either precipitate or protect from the development of scleroderma renal crisis. Arthritis Rheum 1998;41:1613–9.
18. Rodnan GP. The natural history of progressive systemic sclerosis (diffuse scleroderma). Bull Rheum Dis 1963;13:301–4.
19. Rodnan GP. The nature of joint involvement in progressive systemic sclerosis (diffuse scleroderma). Ann Intern Med 1962;56:422–39.
20. Wilson RJ, Rodnan GP, Robin ED. An early pulmonary physiologic abnormality in progressive systemic sclerosis (diffuse scleroderma). Am J Med 1964;36:361–9.
21. Salerni R, Rodnan GP, Leon DF, et al. Pulmonary hypertension in the CREST syndrome variant of progressive systemic sclerosis (scleroderma). Ann Intern Med 1977;86:394–9.
22. Rodnan GP, Fennell RH Jr. Progressive systemic sclerosis sine scleroderma. JAMA 1962;180:665–70.
23. Hayes RL, Rodnan GP. The ultrastructure of skin in progressive systemic sclerosis (scleroderma). I. Dermal collagen fibers. Am J Pathol 1971;63:433–42.
24. Rodnan GP, Myerowitz RL, Justh GO. Morphologic changes in the digital arteries of patients with progressive systemic sclerosis (scleroderma) and Raynaud phenomenon. Medicine (Baltim) 1980;59:393–408.
25. Traub YM, Shapiro AP, Rodnan GP, et al. Hypertension and renal failure (scleroderma renal crisis) in progressive systemic sclerosis. Review of a 25-year experience with 68 cases. Medicine (Baltim) 1983;62:335–52.
26. Rothfield NF, Rodnan GP. Serum antinuclear antibodies in progressive systemic sclerosis (scleroderma). Arthritis Rheum 1968;11:607–17.
27. American Rheumatism Association: Current Topics in Rheumatology. Systemic Sclerosis (Scleroderma): Proceedings of the International Conference on Progressive Systemic Sclerosis held October 20-23, 1981, Austin, Texas. Gower Medical Publishing Ltd., New York, 1985; Black Carol M and Myers Allen R (editors).
28. Kuwana M, Medsger TA Jr. Clinical Aspects of Autoantibodies. Chapter 13 in Scleroderma : From pathogenesis to comprehensive management. New York, NY: Springer Internatio+nal Publishing; 2016. p. 207–20.
29. Steen VD. Autoantibodies in systemic sclerosis. Semin Arthritis Rheum 2005;35: 35–42.
30. Medsger TA Jr, Benedek TG. History of skin thickness assessment and the Rodnan skin thickness scoring method in systemic sclerosis. J Scleroderma Relat Disord 2019;4:83–8.
31. Rodnan GP, Lipinski E, Luksick J. Skin thickness and collagen content in progressive systemic sclerosis and localized scleroderma. Arthritis Rheum 1979;22:130–40.
32. Clements PJ, Lachenbruch PA, Seibold JR, et al. Skin thickness score in systemic sclerosis: an assessment of interobserver variability in 3 independent studies. J Rheumatol 1993;20:1892–6.
33. Clements PJ, Lachenbruch PA, Seibold JR, et al. Inter and intraobserver variability of total skin thickness score (modified Rodnan TSS) in systemic sclerosis. J Rheumatol 1995;22:1281–5.
34. Shulman LE. Diffuse fasciitis with eosinophilia: a new syndrome? Trans Assoc Am Physicians 1975;88:70–86.
35. Barnes L, Rodnan GP, Medsger TA, et al. Short. Eosinophilic fasciitis. A pathologic study of twenty cases. Am J Pathol 1979;96:493–518.

E Carwile LeRoy, MD

Richard M. Silver, MD

KEYWORDS

- Systemic sclerosis (SSc) • Scleroderma • Raynaud phenomenon
- Medical University of South Carolina

KEY POINTS

- E. Carwile LeRoy was one of the pioneers in the study of systemic sclerosis (SSc, scleroderma).
- LeRoy's seminal demonstration of excess collagen synthesis by scleroderma fibroblasts set the stage for future studies elucidating the mechanisms of fibroblast activation.
- LeRoy's enduring legacy rests with his mentees and protoges who continue his quest to unravel the mystery of systemic sclerosis (SSc, scleroderma).

EARLY LIFE

Edward Carwile LeRoy, the second son of prominent Eastern North Carolina attorney John Henry LeRoy and Virginia-native Grace Brown Carwile, was born on January 19, 1933, in Elizabeth City, NC (**Fig. 1**). Carwile excelled scholastically and athletically at football and basketball. His older brother Jack taught Carwile to sail in the local waters, something that would become a lifelong pursuit. When it came time for the senior year of high school, Carwile had completed all but one course the local school had to offer, so he went off to Fork Union Military Academy in Fork Union, VA, where he graduated at the head of his class.

Carwile matriculated at Wake Forest College (now Wake Forest University [WFU]) in 1951. Majoring in science with a minor in English, he excelled in the classroom, was inducted into Phi Beta Kappa, and graduated *summa cum laude*. When not studying, Carwile found time for numerous extracurricular activities, including membership on the college debate team that finished second in the nation his senior year. His debating skills would later serve him well when he would parry with Gerry Rodnan, Larry Shulman, and other notable experts on topics pertaining to pathogenesis and treatment of scleroderma. He served as the president of his fraternity and enjoyed great success in intramural athletics. While at WFU, Carwile met Dee Hughes, who also hailed from Eastern NC, but it would be several more years and on another continent before their courtship would blossom.

Division of Rheumatology & Immunology, Medical University of South Carolina, 96 Jonathan Lucas Street, Suite 822, Charleston, SC 29425, USA
E-mail address: silverr@musc.edu

Rheum Dis Clin N Am 50 (2024) 33–45
https://doi.org/10.1016/j.rdc.2023.08.003
0889-857X/24/© 2023 Elsevier Inc. All rights reserved.

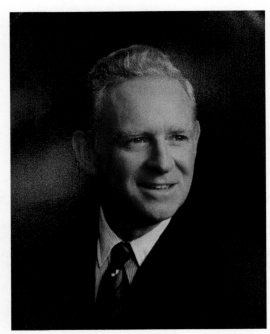

Fig. 1. E. Carwile LeRoy, MD, 1933–2002. (Credit line: Compliments of the LeRoy family.)

Medical Education, Training, and Early Career

Carwile initially had planned to attend medical school in Philadelphia but changed his plans when the University of North Carolina offered him one of the newly inaugurated John Motley Morehead Scholarships. Between his second and third years of medical school, Carwile took a year off for research and earned a Master's degree. Carwile's mentor for his Master's thesis was Dr Kenneth Merle Brinkhous (1908–2000), a pioneer in coagulation and the discoverer of Factor VIII and its absence in patients with hemophilia. Brinkhous was an outstanding mentor who combined friendship and personal concern with a demand for persistent, intense effort. No doubt, Brinkhous found young Carwile up to his standards. Under his mentorship, Carwile published three papers on various aspects of blood platelets and plasma coagulability.[1-3] The mentorship provided by Brinkhous would prove to be pivotal for Carwile's future interest in scleroderma, a disease in which platelets and platelet-derived growth factors (PDGFs) play important roles.

In his senior year of medical school Carwile was elected the President of the Alpha Omega Alpha Honor Medical Society and the Whitehead Society (the medical student body). It was also in his senior year of medical school that Carwile began a courtship with Dee Hughes, whom he knew from his undergraduate school days at WFU. Carwile had been invited to accompany Dr Brinkhous to Paris for the presentation of a research paper. At the same time, Dee was studying in France. Their courtship began in Paris and continued until Dee returned to the states, and they were married on June 11, 1960 (**Fig. 2**).

The newlywed couple made the move from North Carolina to New York City, where Carwile completed his internship and assistant resident year at the Presbyterian Hospital, Columbia-Presbyterian Medical Center. There, Carwile met Dr Charles Christian,

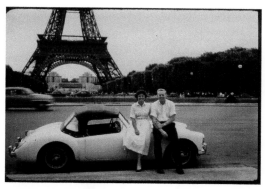

Fig. 2. Carwile with his future bride, Dee, in Paris; ca 1959. (Credit line: Compliments of the LeRoy family.)

the second influential person in Carwile's early medical career. As was often the case in the 1960s, aspiring clinician scientists often would opt for additional training at the National Institutes of Health (NIH) as members of the Public Health Service (PHS) rather than serving as a medical officer in the armed forces. Carwile followed such a path and for the next 3 years worked as a Clinical Associate at the Heart Institute of the NIH. There, he worked closely with Dr Albert Sjoerdsma, who would become the third mentor of Carwile's medical and scientific career. During his years at the NIH and under the mentorship of Dr Sjoerdsma, Carwile's research focused on collagen metabolism. Together with Dr Edward (Ted) Harris, Carwile developed a radioactive hydroxyproline assay for urine and tissues,[4] and he reported on the aggregation of platelets by collagen.[5] On completion of his PHS obligation and NIH training, Carwile returned to Columbia University, College of Physicians and Surgeons, setting up his research laboratory and learning much from another mentor, Dr Charles (Chuck) Christian (**Fig. 3**).

In 1969, Dr Christian moved to the Cornell Medical College and Hospital for Special Surgery, and Carwile was named the Director of the Faulkner Arthritis Center at Columbia Presbyterian Hospital. There, his interest in scleroderma came about somewhat by accident when a friend called Carwile to inquire about an uncle who had recently been diagnosed with scleroderma. While at Columbia, Carwile applied techniques he learned at the NIH and applied them to the study of scleroderma. He published two seminal papers during his time at Columbia, demonstrating for the first time that cultured dermal fibroblasts from patients with scleroderma synthesized and secreted an excess amount of collagen (**Fig. 4, Table 1**).

Working with Dr Hildegard Maricq, whom he recruited to Columbia, Carwile was also among the first to report on differing patterns of capillary morphology seen in connective tissue disease patients.[8] This would be the beginning of his career-long focus on the vascular aspects of scleroderma.

Returning South to Establish a New Program

The LeRoy family, which had grown to include a daughter (DeFord, age 12) and a son (Carwile, Jr, age 10) moved to Charleston, SC, in 1975, when Carwile was recruited to create a Division of Rheumatology & Immunology at the Medical University of South Carolina (MUSC) (**Fig. 5**).

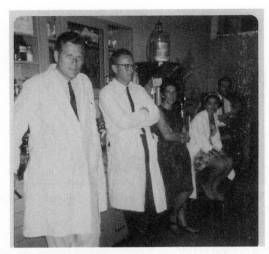

Fig. 3. Dr Carwile LeRoy (*center*) with Dr Charles Christian (*foreground*) and others in the Faulkner Arthritis Center at Columbia Presbyterian Hospital. (Credit line: Compliments of the LeRoy family.)

Before that time, there had been only a single rheumatologist at MUSC, Dr Walter Bonner, the first rheumatologist to practice in the state of South Carolina. The move to the South would not have occurred without the influence of Dr Joe Ross, Chairman of the Department of Medicine, and Dr James W Colbert, MUSCs first Vice-President for Academic Affairs. Dr Colbert was influential in recruiting Carwile and other NIH-trained physician–scientists to lead various divisions and departments at a time when MUSC was beginning to add research to its established clinical expertise. Of note, the youngest child of the late Dr Colbert is the American comedian, writer,

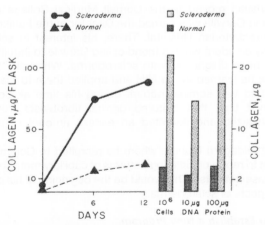

Fig. 4. Experiment demonstrating increased collagen synthesis in vitro by scleroderma skin fibroblasts compared with normal skin fibroblasts. (E. Carwile LeRoy, Increased Collagen Synthesis by Scleroderma Skin Fibroblasts In Vitro A POSSIBLE DEFECT IN THE REGULATION OR ACTIVATION OF THE SCLERODERMA FIBROBLAST. J Clin Invest. 1974;54(4):880–889. https://doi.org/10.1172/JCI107827. © 1974 The American Society for Clinical Investigation.)

Table 1
Selected publications by Dr E Carwile LeRoy and colleagues

Year, Authors	Title	Citation
LeRoy et al,[4] 1966	A modified method for radioactive hydroxyproline assay in urine and tissues after labeled proline administration.	Anal Biochem. 1966;17:377–382
LeRoy,[6] 1972	Connective tissue synthesis by scleroderma skin fibroblasts in cell culture.	J Exp Med. 1972;135:1351–1362
Maricq & LeRoy,[8] 1973	Patterns of finger capillary abnormalities in connective tissue disease by "wide-field" microscopy.	Arthritis Rheum. 1973;16:619–628
LeRoy,[7] 1974	Increased collagen synthesis by scleroderma skin fibroblasts in vitro.	J Clin Invest. 1974;54:880–889
Cannon et al,[9] 1974	The relationship of hypertension and renal failure in scleroderma (progressive systemic sclerosis) to structural and functional abnormalities of the renal cortical circulation.	Medicine. 1974;53:1–46
Kahaleh et al,[10] 1979	Endothelial injury in scleroderma	J Exp Med. 1979;149:1326–1335
Whitman et al,[11] 1982	Variable response to oral angiotensin-converting-enzyme blockade in hypertensive scleroderma patients.	Arthritis Rheum. 1982;25:241–248
Silver et al,[12] 1984	Interstitial lung disease in scleroderma: Analysis by bronchoalveolar lavage.	Arthritis Rheum. 1984;27:1254–1262
Takehara et al,[13] 1987	TGF-β inhibition of endothelial cell proliferation: alteration of epidermal growth factor (EGF) binding and EGF-induced growth regulatory (competence) gene expression.	Cell. 1987;49:415–422
LeRoy & Medsger,[14] 2001	Criteria for the classification of early systemic sclerosis.	J Rheumatol. 2001;28:1573–1576

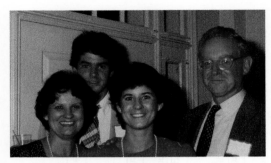

Fig. 5. The LeRoy family in Charleston, SC, 1984. Dee, Carwile, Jr, DeFord, and Carwile (*left to right*). (Credit line: Compliments of the LeRoy family.)

and television host Stephen Colbert. Stephen was a high school classmate and remains a close friend of Carwile, Jr.

Life in Charleston was different from the New Jersey suburbs, and Dee was pleased with the prospect of raising her children in the South, where both she and Carwile were born and raised. Soon, the children adapted to Southern mores (eg, Carwile, Jr added football to his passion for soccer, later helping his high school team win a state championship in soccer, whereas DeFord learned to appreciate single-sex education at Ashley Hall). Dee created a welcoming home for all, first at a Colonial Street residence followed by a move to an historic home on 75 Tradd Street, the former manse of First (Scots) Presbyterian Church. A strong interest in history led Dee to be involved in the Historic Charleston Foundation, becoming a tour guide for the City of Charleston (fluent in French, she was sometimes called on to provide tours for non-English speaking French visitors). Living in a coastal city, Carwile continued to enjoy time for sailing, a passion he handed down to son Carwile, Jr (**Fig. 6**).

Building a Vibrant Rheumatology Program

Carwile set out to build a Rheumatology Division that would become internationally renowned for its studies of scleroderma and Raynaud phenomenon (RP). Dr Hildegard Maricq, who accompanied Carwile on his move from Columbia, established her research laboratory at MUSC and began studies on RP and its relationship to connective tissue diseases. Maricq would devote the next 3 decades to research on microvascular disease and RP in scleroderma. She pioneered the use of widefield microscopy to characterize the microvasculature in primary and secondary RP, a technique that has evolved to current day video capillary microscopy used worldwide. In an important prospective study subsequently confirmed by others, Maricq and LeRoy along with other members of the Division demonstrated that abnormalities in capillary morphology are strongly predictive for the evolution to scleroderma.[15–17] Over the years, postdoctoral fellows would come from elsewhere in the United States, Europe, and South and Central America to work with Hildegard and to learn the technique of nailfold capillary microscopy.

Dr Hendricks H (Hal) Whitman III was one of the US physicians who visited and worked with Maricq and LeRoy. In 1978, just a day after returning to New York City from a 6-week stay in the Maricq laboratory, Hal would end up making an unscheduled return trip to Charleston. At Cornell Medical College, he was working with Dr John H Laragh, a pioneer in the study of the renin–angiotensin system and hypertension, on the development of a new class of antihypertensive agents. Just at that time, a patient

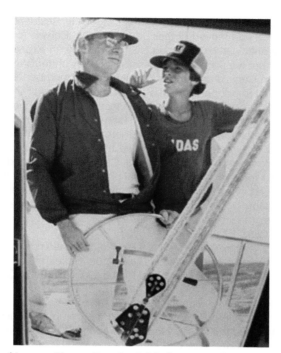

Fig. 6. Carwile as skipper with son Carwile, Jr his first mate. (Credit Line: Complements of the LeRoy family.)

had been admitted to the Medical University Hospital in Charleston and found to be suffering from scleroderma renal crisis; arrangements were hastily made for Hal to return to Charleston and deliver the new angiotensin-converting inhibitor (captopril) to the patient who was now in intensive care. The patient was comatose and had presented with hypertensive retinopathy and failing kidneys. As fate would have it, the Charleston airport was closed that night due to fog, so Hal's plane was diverted to Savannah, GA. From there, he rented a car and drove the 100 miles to Charleston when, well after midnight, he and Carwile along with two rheumatology fellows (Dr Gary Botstein and Dr Frank Harper) administered the captopril to the patient via nasogastric tube. Within minutes, the patient's blood pressure returned to normal in what Dr Gary Botstein recalls as "one of the most rapid/dramatic medical responses I've ever seen." Gary would go on to follow the patient, who recovered normal renal function with well-controlled hypertension, in the MUSC Rheumatology Clinic over the course of his Fellowship and junior faculty appointment.

Leading and Mentoring

Carwile expanded his interest in and studies of scleroderma, recruiting faculty and training fellows who would conduct clinical and basic research while providing rheumatologic care in both in-patient and out-patient settings. Early investigations would demonstrate the heterogeneity of dermal fibroblasts that then led to studies of cellular and serologic factors important for fibroblast activation and endothelial cell injury. Joseph (Joe) Korn was the first to complete the new Rheumatology Fellowship training program at MUSC. While at Columbia, Joe had worked in Carwile's laboratory as a medical student. On completion of his Internal Medicine Residency at University of North Carolina (UNC), Joe moved further South to rejoin Carwile (credit to Joe's wife, Paulette, who only anticipated 3 years in NC followed by an expected return to New York City (NYC), for her support of Joe's passion to study under Carwile's mentorship). With mentoring from Carwile and another young faculty member, Dr Perry Halushka, Joe published his first important work in a paper in the *Journal of Clinical Investigation* describing mononuclear cell modulation of connective tissue function.[18] Shortly thereafter, Joe returned to the Northeast to join Dr Naomi Rothfield's program at the University of Connecticut. Later Joe would move to Boston University (BU) to succeed Dr Alan Cohen as the Division Director. Joe developed his own vibrant and world-renowned program for scleroderma at BU. He was one of Carwile's earliest and most successful trainees and a major force in scleroderma until his untimely death in 2005.

Dr Gary Grotendorst was recruited to the faculty in 1984. During his 3-year tenure as an Assistant Professor, Dr Grotendorst conducted important studies on the chemotactic activity of growth factors and discovered a novel growth factor, connective tissue growth factor (CCN2)[19] (**Fig. 7**).

Gary departed for the University of South Florida, and then moved to the University of Miami. He later moved to the Lovelace Respiratory Research Institute in Albuquerque, NM, where he served as the Director of the Lovelace CounterACT Research Center of Excellence.

Dr Bashar Kahaleh was another early trainee at MUSC who would go on to establish his own independent scleroderma program. After completing his Rheumatology Fellowship, Bashar joined the MUSC faculty and continued his research with Carwile. Together, they demonstrated elevated levels of Factor VIII and increased von Willebrand factor (vWF) activity in the plasma of patients with RP and scleroderma.[20] Carwile would often refer to vWF as a "vascular sed rate." This would be the beginning of Bashar's sustained interest in endothelial cell injury and its role in the pathogenesis of scleroderma. Bashar was recruited to the University of Toledo (formerly the Medical College of Ohio), where he continues to serve as the Chief of the Division of Rheumatology and Immunology.

Notable among these trainees, who would make important scientific contributions and play important leadership roles, is Maria Trojanowska, PhD. Maria completed her postdoctoral fellowship and stayed on as a member of the Division faculty, where

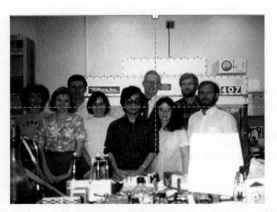

Fig. 7. Research members in the Division of Rheumatology & Immunology at the Medical University of South Carolina. Maria Trojanowska (*fourth from left*); Kazuhiko Takehara (*fifth from left*); Carwile LeRoy (*back, center*); Gary Grotendorst (*far right*).

she was among the first to report on the important effects growth factors and cyto-kines, for example, PDGF and transforming growth factor-beta (TGF-ß) have on dermal fibroblasts from patients with scleroderma.[21,22] Maria established her own successful and well-funded research laboratory at MUSC, where she also mentored numerous aspiring postdoctoral fellows, many of whom would go on to have their own successful and independent research careers. Given her success in research and skills in mentoring, Maria was highly sought after and was recruited to direct the Arthritis & Autoimmune Diseases Research Center at BU Chobanian & Avedisian School of Medicine (**Fig. 8**).

Other trainees would go on to become the Fellowship Program Directors in the United States, including Leslie Staudt, MD (UT-San Antonio), JoAnn Allen, MD (West Virginia University), and Marcy Bolster, MD (MUSC and later Massachusetts General Hospital).

An important feature of the MUSC Scleroderma Program founded by Carwile has been its strong attraction for postdoctoral trainees from around the world who come to Charleston to be mentored in research in scleroderma.

Many bright young physicians and scientists would spend 2 to 3 years at MUSC, working with Carwile and other members of the faculty on cellular and molecular biology of scleroderma fibroblasts. Dr Patricia Carreira and Dr Jose Pablos would go on to successful careers and leadership positions at the Hospital 12 de Octubre in Madrid, Spain. Dr Armando Gabrielli went on to direct the Internal Medicine program at the University of Ancona in Ancona, Italy. Another Italian physician–scientist, Dr Marco Matucci-Cerinic, became a professor at the University of Florence in Florence, Italy, and a world leader in scleroderma. Marco played an instrumental role in the formation of the European Scleroderma Trials and Research Group and is one of the founding members of the World Scleroderma Foundation.

A unique association developed with young physician–scientists who would come to MUSC from Japan to learn and work on scleroderma, many of whom would go on to hold prestigious positions at various medical institutions in their homeland. Kazu-hiko (Kazu) Takehara, MD, was the first of the Japanese postdoctoral fellows to come to Charleston to work in Carwile's Division (**Fig. 9**).

Kazu was later appointed Chairman of the Department of Dermatology at Kanazawa University, where he continued to conduct research on scleroderma and other con-nective tissue diseases until his retirement (**Fig. 10**).

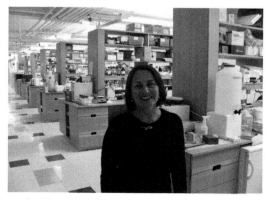

Fig. 8. Maria Trojanowska, PhD, one of Dr LeRoy's early mentees, in her laboratory at Boston University Chobanian & Avedisian School of Medicine where she serves as the Director of the Arthritis & Autoimmune Center.

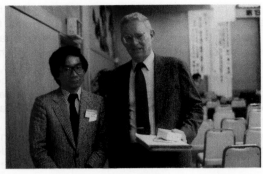

Fig. 9. Dr Kazuhiko Takehara (*left*), the first postdoctoral fellow from Japan to train at MUSC, welcomes Carwile on a visit to Japan.

Other Japanese postdoctoral fellows would become prominent leaders in their respective departments, including Dr Osamu Ishikawa (Chairman, Department of Dermatology, Gunma University), Dr Hironubi Ihn (Professor, Department of Dermatology, Kumamoto University), Dr Tamaki Takeshi (Chairman of Dermatology, International Medical Center of Japan), among others. In all, more than a dozen physician–scientists came from Japan to train at MUSC, most of whom established their own independent research laboratories on returning to Japan.

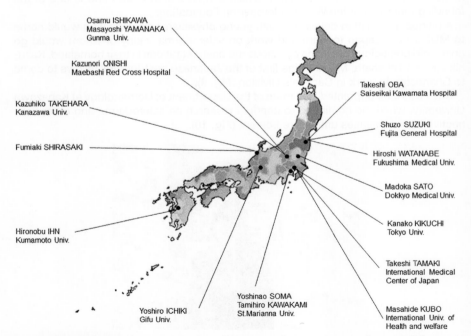

Fig. 10. Map showing the location and affiliations of the many postdoctoral fellows returned to Japan following postdoctoral training in Dr LeRoy's Division of Rheumatology & Immunology at MUSC.

Professional Contributions

Beyond the significant contributions made in scleroderma, Carwile was a born leader who was an active participant in many professional and civic organizations. In the realm of rheumatology, he was a member, fellow, master, committee chair, and officer for the American Rheumatism Association (forerunner of the American College of Rheumatology). He was a member, fellow, and chair of the Rheumatology Subcommittee for the American College of Physicians. Other notable medical society memberships include the Harvey Society, the American Association of Immunologists, the American Federation for Clinical Research, the Southern Society for Clinical Investigation, and the American Osler Society. As a senior faculty member, Carwile led numerous committees for the Department of Medicine, College of Medicine, and for the MUSC. In 2001, MUSCs Board of Trustees recognized Carwile for his many years of service and scientific achievements, bestowing on him the highest University rank of Distinguished University Professor. Carwile also found time to participate in and lead numerous other professional and civic organizations. He received Distinguished Alumni Service Awards from both WFU and UNC.

Ambassador for Scleroderma

Carwile was an enthusiastic roving ambassador for rheumatology and particularly for scleroderma. Over the course of his career, Carwile was an invited speaker and visiting professor at medical schools and professional meetings in 30 states plus the District of Columbia. As a lecturer and educator, he spoke and taught in 18 other countries spanning 5 continents. During a brief vacation in Ancona, Italy, following a speaking engagement in L'Aquila, Carwile suffered a fatal cerebrovascular event. This sad and unexpected event shook the rheumatology world and dealt a great blow to the international scleroderma community.

Personal Reflections

After completing a Fellowship in Rheumatology at the University of California-San Diego (UCSD), Carwile offered me my first faculty appointment in the MUSCs Division of Rheumatology & Immunology. The appointment was facilitated by a telephone call (long before email) to Carwile by my program director and chief at UCSD, Dr Nathan Zvaifler. The appointment and subsequent move to Charleston was received with great appreciation, especially because my wife was a native of Charleston and was eager to return home. The LeRoys provided a most gracious welcome to this young couple, as they did for all new members and visitors to the Division (**Fig. 11**).

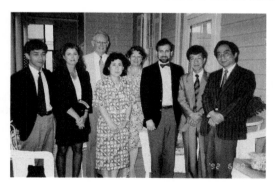

Fig. 11. On the veranda at the LeRoy home on 75 Tradd Street. Dr and Mrs LeRoy with Dr and Mrs Rick Silver, Dr.Kazu Takehara (*far right*), and visiting physicians from the Gifu University Medical School, 1992.

The LeRoy home on Tradd Street was the scene of many enjoyable social and professional events, including journal clubs held on the veranda where the choir from next door First (Scots) Presbyterian Church could often be heard.

Carwile was supportive of my initial attempts to establish a laboratory and continue the research on rheumatoid synovial lymphocytes begun in my fellowship. It soon dawned on me, however, that I needed to take advantage of the rich patient population and research environment and focus instead on scleroderma. I chose to study scleroderma-associated interstitial lung disease (ILD), and my timing was fortuitous as the angiotensin-converting enzyme inhibitor, captopril, had recently been developed to treat scleroderma renal crisis,[10] making ILD an even more important complication of the disease. This has remained my research focus for nearly 4 decades, and I am indebted to Carwile for his early support and inspiration. Indeed, a notable aspect of Carwile's legacy is his interest and support for young investigators who came from far and wide to work in the Division at MUSC.

In late 1995, Carwile was named Chairman of MUSCs Department of Microbiology and Immunology, at which time I was appointed to replace him as the Director of the Division of Rheumatology & Immunology, a position I held until 2018. During my 23-year tenure as the Director, the Division saw significant growth in clinical and research productivity. Carwile deserves much credit for the success that the Division achieved following his departure. As stated by Sir Isaac Newton, *If I have seen further it is by standing on the shoulders of giants*. During my tenure as the Division Director, we maintained a focus on scleroderma and other connective tissue diseases, enlarging our research portfolio with the recruitment of Dr Gary Gilkeson and Dr Jim Oates (lupus), Dr Carol Feghali-Bostwick (scleroderma), Dr Betty Tsao (genetic risk factors for autoimmune diseases), and several other important clinical and research faculty. As I wrote in my memoriam paraphrasing an epithet to one of Carwile's heroes, Sir William Osler, "'Men are immortalized on this earth when their good actions and qualities are imitated by those who come after'. So it has been with Dr LeRoy. So let it be with us."[23]

ACKNOWLEDGMENTS

The author gratefully acknowledges the LeRoy family—Dee, DeFord, and Carwile, Jr—for their review of the article and for permission to publish family photographs.

REFERENCES

1. Brinkhous KM, LeRoy EC, Cornell WP, et al. Macroscopic studies of platelet agglutination: nature of thrombocyte agglutinating activity of plasma. Proc Soc Exp Biol Med 1958;98:37–383.
2. Mason RG, LeRoy EC, Brinkhous KM. Cation specificity of thrombocyte agglutinating activity (Tag) of canine plasma. Proc Soc Exp Biol Med 1959;102:253–5.
3. LeRoy EC, Mason RG, Brinkhous KM. Species differences in platelet agglutination in man and in the dog, swine and rabbit. Am J Physiol 1960;199:183–6.
4. LeRoy EC, Harris ED, Sjoerdsma A. A modified procedure for radioactive hydroxyproline assay in urine and tissues after labeled proline administration. Anal Biochem 1966;17:377–82.
5. Wilner GD, Nossel HI, LeRoy EC. Aggregation of platelets by collagen. J Clin Invest 1968;47:2616–21.
6. LeRoy EC. Connective tissue synthesis by scleroderma skin fibroblasts in cell culture. J Exp Med 1972;135:1351–62.

7. LeRoy EC. Increased collagen synthesis by scleroderma skin fibroblasts in vitro. J Clin Invest 1974;54:880–9.
8. Maricq HR, LeRoy EC. Patterns of finger capillary abnormalities in connective tissue disease by "wide-field" microscopy. Arthritis Rheum 1973;16:619–28.
9. Cannon PJ, Hassar M, Case DB, et al. The relationship of hypertension and renal failure in scleroderma (progressive systemic sclerosis) to structural and functional abnormalities of the renal cortical circulation. Medicine 1974;53:1–46.
10. Kahaleh MB, Sherer GK, LeRoy EC. Endothelial injury in scleroderma. J Exp Med 1979;149:1326–35.
11. Whitman HH III, Case DB, Laragh JH, et al. Variable response to oral angiotensin-converting-enzyme blockade in hypertensive scleroderma patients. Arthritis Rheum 1982;25:241–8.
12. Silver RM, Metcalf J, Stanley JH, et al. Interstitial lung disease in scleroderma: analysis by bronchoalveolar lavage. Arthritis Rheum 1984;27:1254–62.
13. Takehara K, LeRoy EC, Grotendorst GR. TGF-ß inhibition of endothelial cell proliferation: alteration of EGF binding and EGF-induced growth regulatory (competence) gene expression. Cell 1987;49:415–22.
14. LeRoy EC, Medsger TA Jr. Criteria for the classification of early systemic sclerosis. J Rheumatol 2001;28:1573–6.
15. Harper FE, Maricq HR, Turner RE, et al. A prospective study of Raynaud's phenomenon and early connective tissue disease. Am J Med 1982;72:883–8.
16. Maricq HR, Weinberger AB, LeRoy EC. Early detection of scleroderma-spectrum disorders by in vivo capillary microscopy: a prospective study of patients with Raynaud's phenomenon. J Rheumatol 1982;9:289–91.
17. Maricq HR, Harper EF, Khan MM, et al. Microvascular abnormalities as possible predictors of disease subsets in Raynaud's phenomenon and early connective tissue disease. Clin Exp Rheum 1983;1:195–205.
18. Korn JH, Halushka PV, LeRoy EC. Mononuclear cell modulation of connective tissue function. J Clin Invest 1980;65:543–54.
19. Bradham DM, Igarashi A, Potter RL, et al. Connective tissue growth factor: a cysteine-rich mitogen secreted by human vascular endothelial cells is related to the SRC-induced immediate early gene product CEF-10. J Cell Biol 1991; 113:1285–94.
20. Kahaleh MB, Osborn I, LeRoy EC. Increased factor VIII/von Willebrand factor antigen and von Willebrand factor activity in scleroderma and Raynaud's phenomenon. Ann Intern Med 1981;94:482–4.
21. Yamakage A, Kikuchi K, Smith EA, et al. Selective upregulation of platelet-derived growth factor-alpha receptors by transforming growth factor ß in scleroderma fibroblasts. J Exp Med 1992;175:1227–34.
22. Kikuchi K, Hartl CW, Smith EA, et al. Direct demonstration of transcriptional activation of collagen gene expression in systemic sclerosis fibroblasts: insensitivity to TGFß1 stimulation. BBRC (Biochem Biophys Res Commun) 1992;187:45–50.
23. Silver RM. In memoriam: E. Carwile LeRoy, MD, 1933-2002. Arthritis Rheum 2002; 46:2564.

Charles L Christian
Model Physician Scientist and Mentor

Mary K. Crow, MD*, Josef S. Smolen, MD

KEYWORDS

- Rheumatoid arthritis • Systemic lupus erythematosus • Vasculitis • HSS

RHEUMATOID ARTHRITIS

Dr Christian's research addressing immunologic mechanisms in rheumatoid arthritis (RA) was inspired by Dr Ragan, who with Dr Harry M. Rose can be credited with the discovery of rheumatoid factor (**Table 1**). Dr Ragan was Chairman of the Department of Medicine at Columbia University College of Physicians & Surgeons at the time Chuck joined their faculty as a young physician. In 1957, in a paper published with Dr Ragan, and in a single-author study published in *Journal of Experimental Medicine*, Chuck described aggregated gamma globulin as the serum target of rheumatoid factor.[4] This study was only the first of many that would provide a detailed characterization of the autoantibodies and immune complexes that are essential mediators of autoimmune rheumatic diseases.

Chuck's thinking was systematic. When in 1961 (as an Instructor at Columbia) he asked himself how rheumatoid factor might be related to RA, he articulated 3 hypotheses: (1) as a non-specific reflection of synovitis or vasculitis, (2) as a pathogenic mediator of the disease, or (3) as a response to the agent driving the disease but not itself contributing to disease pathogenesis.[18] He favored the third. When in 1964 he discussed evidence that the immune system was involved in the pathogenesis of rheumatic disease, he laid out the case point by point and then described two hypotheses for its action: direct antibody-mediated injury versus injury due to antigen-antibody reactions, drawing the analogy to serum sickness.[19] At that time, knowledge of the cellular arm of the immune system was more limited than knowledge of antibodies and their pathogenic potential, but with the information at hand, Chuck went on to demonstrate the role of immune complexes and consistently showed breadth of both clinical and scientific knowledge, a logical thought process, and a dispassionate assessment of potential mechanisms of disease.

SYSTEMIC LUPUS ERYTHEMATOSUS

Patients with systemic lupus erythematosus (SLE) were diagnosed and managed by Chuck throughout his career, first at Columbia, for 25 years at Hospital for Special

Mary Kirkland Center for Lupus Research, Hospital for Special Surgery, New York, NY 10021, USA
* Corresponding author.
E-mail address: crowm@hss.edu

Rheum Dis Clin N Am 50 (2024) 47–55
https://doi.org/10.1016/j.rdc.2023.09.002
0889-857X/24/© 2023 Published by Elsevier Inc.

rheumatic.theclinics.com

Table 1
Charles L Christian, MD: major scientific contributions

Observation	References
Identification of aggregated gamma globulin as the target of rheumatoid factor	1,2
Demonstration of the specificity of anti-DNA antibodies for a diagnosis of SLE	3
Association of anti-DNA antibodies with complement components	4,5
Application of anti-DNA antibodies as a biomarker of lupus disease activity	6
Demonstration of the role of immune complexes in chronic glomerulonephritis	7–9
Description of the natural history of SLE	10
Support for a genetic contribution to SLE based on studies of monozygotic and dizygotic twins	11-13
Demonstration of presence of hepatitis B 'Australia' antigen in immune complexes from patients with polyarteritis nodosa	14-16
High- dose methylprednisolone as treatment for SLE	17

Abbreviation: SLE, systemic lupus erythematosus

Surgery (HSS) (**Fig. 1**) and during his 'retirement', when he served as chief of the one-person Division of Rheumatology at the University of Florida in Jacksonville, Florida. Those patients served as inspiration for research studies leading to seminal observations that continue to guide our understanding of the pathophysiology of SLE. After the description of the lupus erythematosus (LE) cell in 1957, there was growing interest in characterizing the plasma factors involved in formation of that characteristic cell.[20–25] In 1958, as a postdoctoral fellow supported by the Arthritis Foundation, Chuck developed a modification of the latex fixation test, coating latex particles with calf thymus nucleoprotein.[3] Characteristic of the experimental rigor Chuck would demonstrate throughout his career, his data nailed the specificity of the identified antibodies for patients with a clinical diagnosis of SLE and those demonstrating the LE cell phenomenon. He later provided extensive analyses of the specificity and biochemical

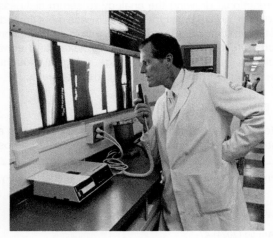

Fig. 1. Charles L Christian, MD, dictating a patient note in the Hospital for Special Surgery arthritis clinic, circa 1980.

properties of anti-DNA antibodies, including their association with complement (shown by Chuck and Jane Morse to be due to C1q) and formation of cryoprecipitates in sera from some lupus patients with active disease.[4,5,26,27] His data supported the hypothesis that immune complexes can mediate tissue injury.[7-9] Chuck's report, with Graham Hughes and Selwyn Cohen, of the relationship between levels of anti-DNA antibodies, best measured using the ammonium sulfate precipitation (Farr) technique, and lupus disease activity, published in *Annals of the Rheumatic Diseases*, was the basis of the proposal that serologic criteria could be used as guides in the management of the patient with SLE (**Fig. 2**).[6]

From Chuck's study of the properties of autoantibodies came a career-long curiosity regarding the composition of immune complexes and their contribution to organ inflammation and damage. He demonstrated that non-precipitating antibody favored the development of chronic glomerulonephritis as well as the role of reticuloendothelial cells in clearing immune complexes, and he proposed that lupus nephritis, whether membranous or proliferative, was driven by deposition of antibody-antigen complexes.[7-9,28]

Laboratory insights were enriched and were guided by Chuck's personal experience diagnosing and managing hundreds of patients with SLE. It was his landmark paper with Dorothy Estes, 'The Natural History of Systemic Lupus Erythematosus by Prospective Analysis,' published in *Medicine* in 1971 that served as the primer on the clinical manifestations and prognostic factors of SLE for several generations of medical students.[10] The value of careful monitoring and clinical and immunologic characterization of monozygotic and dizygotic twins was described in a series of publications that strongly supported a genetic contribution to SLE.[11-13] Autoantibodies and tubuloreticular inclusions, now understood to reflect type I interferon, were seen prior to development of clinical symptoms in 'healthy' twins, while impaired lymphocyte function was associated with, rather than preceded, development of clinical SLE.[13] Together, those observations can be viewed as precursors to a current view that generation of autoantibodies and interferon represent 2 fundamental contributors to SLE pathogenesis.

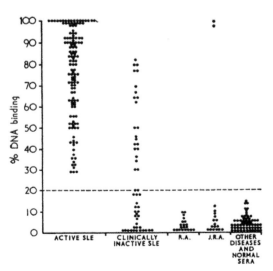

Fig. 2. DNA-binding activity in serum samples from clinically active or inactive patients with SLE. JRA, juvenile rheumatoid arthritis; RA, rheumatoid arthritis; SLE, systemic lupus erythematosu. (Fig. 2 is adapted from Hughes and colleagues[6].)

VASCULITIS

Chuck acknowledged that the insights gleaned from physical examination, imaging, and laboratory investigation were insufficient to fully understand rheumatic diseases and implement optimally effective therapies. He expressed a most compelling question: what provides the stimulus for the immune reaction in autoimmune rheumatic diseases?[19] That curiosity led him to pursue the possibility that the response of the immune system to microbial infection might be at the heart of many of our diseases. The concept was supported by his identification of bacterial protein in immune complexes from a patient with bacterial endocarditis,[29] but the potential for a microbe to serve as a direct participant in an autoimmune rheumatic disease was more speculative.

Chuck's experience in the analysis of antigen-antibody complexes in RA and SLE was a precursor to his studies of immune complexes from patients with polyarteritis nodosa, performed with David Gocke and colleagues[14–16] The 'Australia antigen' had been described in 1965 by Blumberg and colleagues based on observations of an isoprecipitin in sera from patients with hemophilia who had received multiple blood transfusions, and he had documented the antigen on viral-like particles.[30–32] Chuck's study of patients with polyarteritis nodosa documented complexes containing antibody and the Australia antigen.[14] At the time of publication of this work, in *Lancet* in 1970, data had been accumulating that the Australia antigen represented a component of hepatitis B virus, a discovery for which Blumberg was awarded the Nobel Prize in 1976.[32] The data presented by Chuck strongly supported an etiologic role for the hepatitis B virus in the systemic vasculitis seen in the study patients, and he proposed that the clinical syndrome reflected an immunologic response to an infectious agent.[14,15]

A POTENTIAL ROLE FOR VIRUSES

The clinical presentation of SLE or vasculitis often features influenza-like symptoms characteristic of common infections. Data from murine lupus models, particularly the studies of Robert Mellors, who had established a research laboratory at HSS, stimulated Chuck's interest in pursuing a potential viral etiology for SLE.[33] Dr Mellors had demonstrated expression of the glycoprotein gp70 of the non-ecotropic endogenous retrovirus in kidneys from NZB/W F1 lupus mice, now understood to be attributable to a genomic deletion resulting in deficiency of a transcriptional regulator needed for control of endogenous retrovirus transcription.[34] While serologic analyses performed with Paul Phillips demonstrated elevated titers of antibodies specific for several viruses in SLE, the interpretation was that the antibodies represented a polyclonal increase in immunoglobulin rather than a mark of a specific agent.[35–38] The possibility that a virus might serve as a trigger for autoimmune rheumatic disease persists to this day, with current investigation of the host response to severe acute respiratory syndrome coronavirus-2 (SARS-CoV-2) generating a growing number of reports of development of autoantibodies in patients with COVID-19.[39] The observation that a non-structural protein of SARS-CoV-2 can bind to the U1 RNA of the small nuclear ribonucleoprotein (RNP) particle that is the target of anti-RNP antibodies provides a potential mechanism consistent with Chuck's prediction of an etiologic role for a virus in development of systemic autoimmunity.[40]

MENTOR AND ACADEMIC LEADER

Dr Christian's impact on the training of a generation of academic rheumatologists and as a leader in academic medicine equaled his contributions to science. Ironically, his career as a mentor began with his first trainee, Harry Spiera, who developed his own career as a revered clinical rheumatologist in New York City, and ended with his final trainee, Harry's son Robert Spiera, who currently leads studies of novel therapeutics in systemic sclerosis and vasculitis. In early 1970, Chuck was recruited to HSS, where he served as Physician-in-Chief and Director of Rheumatic Diseases, as well as Chief of the Division of Rheumatology at Weill Cornell Medical College from 1970 to 1995. He developed a leading rheumatology fellowship training programme and together with his mentees extended his impact on clinical medicine (**Fig. 3**). With Kimberly and colleagues he introduced high-dose pulse methylprednisolone therapy for patients with lupus nephritis.[17] With Hal Whitman and John Laragh he identified angiotensin-converting enzyme blockade as an effective treatment for scleroderma renal crisis.[41] Impaired Fc-mediated mononuclear phagocyte function in patients with lupus nephritis was documented in studies performed by several HSS rheumatology fellows mentored by Chuck.[42]

The 1970s through the 1980s were a period of growth for rheumatology at HSS. Lawrence Kagen, Robert Lightfoot, Michael Lockshin, and Paul Phillips came to HSS from Columbia and together with Chuck established a strong presence among the orthopedic-focused faculty at the institution. Stellar physician scientists, particularly Bob Kimberly and Robert Inman, joined the faculty following completion of their training. Later, in 1983, Jane Salmon and the author were invited by Chuck to join the faculty, primarily as physician scientists. Stephen Paget, who later succeeded Chuck as HSS Physician-in-Chief, was among those trainees who joined as clinical faculty. graduates of the HSS rheumatology training programme have gone on to serve as chiefs of divisions of rheumatology at academic institutions and as leaders of the American College of Rheumatology (ACR) (John Sergent, Allan Gibofsky, Peggy Crow). International colleagues were particularly welcomed by Chuck, including Graham Hughes and Stefano Bombardieri, who spent time at HSS as visiting scientists or research fellows. Persistence paid off when Keith Elkon finally made his way from London to HSS, where he pursued investigation of some of the autoantibodies initially studied by Chuck.[43] Keith made important contributions to the field of rheumatology and HSS through his own work and as a consequence of his and Chuck's recruitment of Aziz Gharavi, Dror Mevorach, Jorn Drappa, Akshay Vaishnaw, and Eloisa Bonfa, primarily as research trainees. Aziz had worked with Graham Hughes and Keith at Hammersmith Hospital in London where he described anticardiolipin antibodies. He continued his work on the antiphospholipid syndrome and its associated antibodies with Keith and Mike Lockshin at HSS. Dror studied mechanisms of clearance of apoptotic cells with Keith and went on to serve as Chairman of Medicine at the HadassahHebrew University Medical Center in Jerusalem. Both Jorn and Akshay have gone

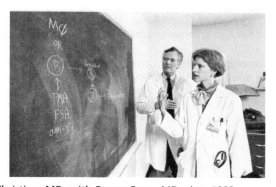

Fig. 3. Charles L Christian, MD, with Peggy Crow, MD, circa 1983.

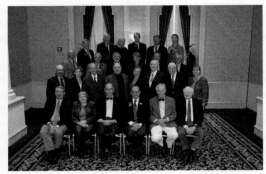

Fig. 4. Charles L Christian, MD, with other past presidents of the American College of Rheumatology and the Rheumatology Research Foundation. Pictured (left to right): Front row— Stanley B Cohen, Lynn Bonfiglio, Stephen E Malawista, David G Borenstein, Charles L Christian and Daniel J McCarty, Jr. Second row—Neal S Birnbaum, Audrey B Uknis, David A Fox, Michael H Weisman, Bevra H Hahn, J Claude Bennett, Evan Calkins and Elizabeth A Tindall. Third row—Michael E Weinblatt, Joseph D Croft, Jr, Allan Gibofsky, Mary K Crow, John S Sergent and Ronald L Kaufman. Fourth row—James R O'Dell, Arthur L Weaver, Shaun Ruddy, Robert F Meenan, William N Kelley and Leslie J Crofford. (Photo courtesy of The Rheumatology Research Foundation.)

on to distinguished careers in biotechnology after studying the Fas mutation in the MRL/lpr lupus model and in patients with the autoimmune lymphoproliferative syndrome with Keith. Eloisa described the role of anti-P autoantibodies in Keith's laboratory and has established a distinguished career as a leader at the University of Sao Paolo Medical School in Brazil. Keith continues to make significant contributions to unraveling the pathogenesis of SLE in his current position at the University of Washington. Chuck's final recruit was Lionel Ivashkiv from Brigham and Women's Hospital. Lionel currently serves as HSS Chief Scientific Officer and has defined cell signaling pathways important in RA. Apologies to the many mentees and collaborators of Chuck who are not mentioned here. Together, we are a family of dedicated rheumatologists who cherish our experiences guided by an incomparable role model.

Commitment to service to the academic community was an important feature of Chuck's career. He twice served as Acting Physician-in-Chief at the New York Hospital and as Acting Chairman of the Department of Medicine at Cornell University Medical College.

He served as Editor-in-Chief of *Arthritis & Rheumatism* from 1971 to 1975, was President of the ACR in 1976 and 1977, and received the Presidential Gold Medal of the ACR in 1996, in recognition of outstanding achievements in rheumatology over an entire career (**Fig. 4**). He was an emeritus member of the American Society for Clinical Investigation.

Chuck was the ultimate 'triple-threat' contributor to academic medicine. But he was more than a creative scientist, skilled clinician, educator, mentor, and leader. He was elegant, kind, generous, and respectful of his colleagues and particularly caring for his patients. There are few rheumatologists who have left such a deep and significant mark on the field or who so perfectly represent what we might all aspire to achieve in our own careers.

CONTRIBUTORS

The author is solely responsible for all aspects of the submitted article.

FUNDING

The authors have not declared a specific grant for this research from any funding agency in the public, commercial or not-for-profit sectors.

PATIENT AND PUBLIC INVOLVEMENT

Patients and/or the public were not involved in the design, conduct, reporting, or dissemination plans of this research.

PATIENT CONSENT FOR PUBLICATION

Not required.

PROVENANCE AND PEER REVIEW

Commissioned; externally peer reviewed.

COMPETING INTERESTS

None declared.

REFERENCES

1. Ragan C, Christian CL. Serologic reactions seen in rheumatoid arthritis. Trans Am Clin Climatol Assoc 1957-1958;69:1–8.
2. Christian CL. Characterization of the reactant (gamma globulin factor) in the F II precipitin reaction and the F II tanned sheep cell agglutination test. J Exp Med 1958;108:139–57.
3. Christian CL, Mendez- Bryan R, Larson DL. Latex agglutination test for disseminated lupus erythematosus. Proc Soc Exp Biol Med 1958;98:820–3.
4. Morse JH, Christian CL. Immunological studies of the 11S protein component of the human complement system. J Exp Med 1964;119:195–209.
5. Hanauer LB, Christian CL. Clinical studies of hemolytic complement and the 11S component. Am J Med 1967;42:882–90.
6. Hughes GR, Cohen SA, Christian CL. Anti- Dna activity in systemic lupus erythematosus. A diagnostic and therapeutic guide. Ann Rheum Dis 1971;30:259–64.
7. Christian CL, Desimone AR, Abruzzo JL. Anti- Dna antibodies in hyperimmunized rabbits. J Exp Med 1965;121:309–21.
8. Pincus T, Haberkern R, Christian CL. Experimental chronic glomerulitis. J Exp Med 1968;127:819–32.
9. Christian CL. Immune- Complex disease. N Engl J Med 1969;280:878–84.
10. Estes D, Christian CL. The natural history of systemic lupus erythematosus by prospective analysis. Medicine 1971;50:85–96.
11. Block SR, Winfield JB, Lockshin MD, et al. Proceedings: twin studies in systemic lupus erythematosus (SLE). Arthritis Rheum 1975;18:285.
12. Block SR, Winfield JB, Lockshin MD, et al. Studies of twins with systemic lupus erythematosus. A review of the literature and presentation of 12 additional sets. Am J Med 1975;59:533–52.
13. Block SR, Lockshin MD, Winfield JB, et al. Immunologic observations on 9 sets of twins either concordant or discordant for SLE. Arthritis Rheum 1976;19:545–54.
14. Gocke DJ, Hsu K, Morgan C, et al. Association between polyarteritis and Australia antigen. Lancet 1970;2:1149–53.

15. Gocke DJ, Hsu K, Morgan C, et al. Vasculitis in association with Australia antigen. J Exp Med 1971;134:330–6.
16. Inman RD, McDougal JS, Redecha PB, et al. Isolation and characterization of circulating immune complexes in patients with hepatitis B systemic vasculitis. Clin Immunol Immunopathol 1981;21:364–74.
17. Kimberly RP, Lockshin MD, Sherman RL, et al. High-Dose intr avenous methyl-prednisolone pulse therapy in systemic lupus erythematosus. Am J Med 1981; 70:817–24.
18. Christian CL. The possible significance of the "rheumatoid factor.". Arthritis Rheum 1961;4:86–8.
19. Christian CL. Rheumatoid arthritis – Etiologic considerations. Arthritis Rheum 1964;7:455–66.
20. Hargraves MM, Richmond H, Morton R. Presentation of two bone marrow elements; the tart cell and the L.E. cell. Proc Staff Meet Mayo Clin 1948;23:25–8.
21. Holman HR, Kunkel HG. Affinity between the lupus erythematosus serum factor and cell nuclei and nucleoprotein. Science 1957;126:162–3.
22. Friou GJ, Finch SC, Detre KD. Interaction of nuclei and globulin from lupus erythematosis serum demonstrated with fluorescent antibody. J Immunol 1958;80: 324–9.
23. Robbins WC, Holman HR, Deicher H, et al. Complement fixation with cell nuclei and DNA in lupus erythematosus. Proc Soc Exp Biol Med 1957;96:575–9.
24. Seligmann M. Mise en évidence dans le sérum de malades atteints de lupus erythémateux disséminé d'une substance déterminant une réaction de précipitation avec l'acide désoxyribonucléique [Demonstration in the blood of patients with disseminated lupus erythematosus a substance determining a precipitation reaction with desoxyribonucleic acid]. C R Hebd Seances Acad Sci 1957;245: 243–5.
25. Miescher P, Strassle R. New serological methods for the detection of the L.E. factor. Vox Sang 1957;2:283–7.
26. Christian CL, Hatfield WB, Chase PH. Systemic lupus erythematosus. cryoprecipitation of sera. J Clin Invest 1963;42:823–9.
27. Hanauer LB, Christian CL. Studies of cryoproteins in systemic lupus erythematosus. J Clin Invest 1967;46:400–8.
28. Seegal BC, Accinni L, Andres GA, et al. Immunologic studies of autoimmune disease in NZB/NZW F1 mice. J Exp Med 1969;130:203–16.
29. Inman RD, Redecha PB, Knechtle SJ, et al. Identification of bacterial antigens in circulating immune complexes of infective endocarditis. J Clin Invest 1982;70: 271–80.
30. Blumberg BS, Alter HJ, VISNICH S. A "New" Antigen in Leukemia Sera. JAMA 1965;191:541–6.
31. Millman I, London WT, Sutnick AI, et al. Australia antigen- antibody complexes. Nature 1970;226:83–4.
32. Bayer ME, Blumberg BS, Werner B. Particles associated with Australia antigen in the sera of patients with leukaemia, Down's syndrome and hepatitis. Nature 1968; 218:1057–9.
33. Mellors RC, Mellors JW. Antigen related to mammalian type- C RNA viral p30 proteins is located in renal glomeruli in human systemic lupus erythematosus. Proc Natl Acad Sci U S A 1976;73:233–7.
34. Treger RS, Pope SD, Kong Y, et al. The lupus susceptibility locus Sgp3 encodes the suppressor of endogenous retrovirus expression SNERV. Immunity 2019;50: 334–47.

35. Phillips PE, Christian CL. Myxovirus antibody increases in human connective tissue disease. Science 1970;168:982–4.
36. Phillips PE, Christian CL. Virus antibodies in systemic lupus erythematosus and other connective tissue diseases. Ann Rheum Dis 1973;32:450–6.
37. Christian CL, Phillips PE. Viruses and autoimmunity. Am J Med 1973;54:611–20.
38. Christian CL. Editorial: systemic lupus erythematosus and type C RNA viruses. N Engl J Med 1976;295:501–2.
39. Chang SE, Feng A, Meng W, et al. New-Onset IgG autoantibodies in hospitalized patients with COVID-19. medRxiv 2021. https://doi.org/10.1101/2021.01.27.21250559 [Epub ahead of print: 29 Jan 2021].
40. Banerjee AK, Blanco MR, Bruce EA, et al. SARS- CoV-2 disrupts splicing, translation, and protein trafficking to suppress host defenses. Cell 2020;183:1325–39.
41. Whitman HH, Case DB, Laragh JH, et al. Variable response to oral angiotensin-converting-enzyme blockade in hypertensive scleroderma patients. Arthritis Rheum 1982;25:241–8.
42. Parris TM, Kimberly RP, Inman RD, et al. Defective Fc receptor-mediated function of the mononuclear phagocyte system in lupus nephritis. Ann Intern Med 1982;97:526–32.
43. Christian CL, Elkon KB. Autoantibodies to intracellular proteins. Clinical and biologic significance. Am J Med 1986;80:53–61.

J. Claude Bennett, MD
Scholar, Physician, and Leader

S. Louis Bridges Jr, MD, PhD[a,b,]*, Steffen Gay, MD[c]

KEYWORDS

- Rheumatology • Internal medicine • Immunoglobulins • J. Claude Bennett
- University of Alabama at Birmingham

KEY POINTS

- During his training and early research career, Dr Bennett studied the molecular basis of antibody formation.
- Dr Bennett led the UAB Division of Clinical Immunology and Rheumatology, and the UAB Department of Microbiology, and had a great impact on the growth of the immunology researcher enterprise at UAB.
- As Chair of the UAB Department of Medicine, Dr Bennett had a substantial impact on post-graduate medical education, patient care, and biomedical research.
- After his term as President of UAB, Dr Bennett returned to identifying ways to better treat patients through his leadership roles at BioCryst Pharmaceuticals.

EARLY CAREER

A native of Birmingham, Alabama, J. Claude Bennett received his undergraduate degree from Howard College (now Samford University) and his MD degree *cum laude* from Harvard Medical School. After completing his housestaff training in Birmingham, Bennett sought research training in the field of arthritis, and more specifically in the field of antibodies. Dr Bennett undertook his postgraduate medical and scientific training at a unique time in history. In 1960, the structure of DNA, the substance of life, had been discovered less than a decade earlier and fundamental questions were being posed. For example, the prevailing one gene-one protein hypothesis posed an interesting paradox. How can this be true if humans can generate millions of antibodies to different antigens?

After his clinical training, Dr Bennett embarked on a fellowship at Massachusetts General Hospital and Harvard Medical School, where he worked with Edgar Haber,

[a] Department of Medicine, Division of Rheumatology, Hospital for Special Surgery, 535 East 70th Street, New York, NY 10021, USA; [b] Division of Rheumatology, Weill Cornell Medicine, Weill Cornell Medical College; [c] Department of Rheumatology, University Hospital Zürich, Rämistrasse 1008091 Zurich, Switzerland
* Corresponding author. Hospital for Special Surgery, 535 East 70th Street, New York, NY 10021.
E-mail address: bridgesl@hss.edu

Rheum Dis Clin N Am 50 (2024) 57–63
https://doi.org/10.1016/j.rdc.2023.08.004
0889-857X/24/© 2023 Elsevier Inc. All rights reserved.

MD, an outstanding molecular scientist and immunochemist.[1] His first paper was published in *PNAS* and was focused on the antigen–antibody interaction.[2] Next, Dr Bennett trained in the Laboratory of Molecular Biology of the National Institute of Arthritis and Metabolic Diseases with William Dreyer. In 1964, Bennett wrote an article on Genetic Coding for Protein Structure in Annual Review of Biochemistry which began "The field encompassed by this review has developed so recently that it has never before been covered in annual review of biochemistry."[3]

Bennett continued to work as a post-doctoral fellow with Dr Dreyer who moved to the California Institute of Technology,[4] and together they focused on concepts of genetic coding for protein structure, gene splicing and monoclonal antibodies. Based on peptide analyses of myeloma proteins, they delineated the constant (C) and variable (V) regions of immunoglobulin molecules.[5] These studies resulted in a general hypothesis for the generation of antibody diversity. In 1965, they published a landmark paper entitled, "The Molecular Basis of Antibody Formation: A Paradox".[6] Drs Bennett and Dreyer were among the first scientists to propose gene segment rearrangements as an explanation for the paradox of the one gene-one protein hypothesis versus the capacity of humans to generate antibodies to millions of different antigens. This article was highlighted on the front page of the New York Times under the headline: "Key to Antibody Origin May be Near".[7] This work led to Bennett's clinical research examining the structures of rheumatoid factors and relationships to various infectious agents as initiators of inflammatory process seen in rheumatoid arthritis.[8] Dr Bennett went on to have a successful research career, with more than 200 scientific publications focused mostly on immunoglobulins, complement, and the phylogenetic development of the immune system.[9]

Leadership at UAB and Nationally

Dr Bennett was recruited to the faculty of UAB in 1965 by Dr Howard Holley, the founder of the UAB Division of Rheumatology (**Fig. 1**). At that time, Dr Bennett had already envisioned the growth and advancement of the fields of rheumatology and immunology. He ascended to the rank of professor in 1970, when he was appointed Chief of the UAB Division of Clinical Immunology and Rheumatology. He held the

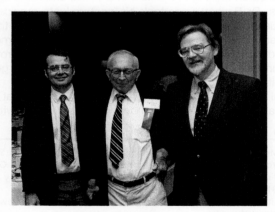

Fig. 1. The first three Directors of the UAB Division of Clinical immunology and Rheumatology, circa 1985. L to R: Bill Koopman, MD (1982–1994), Howard L. Holley, MD, Founding Director, and J. Claude Bennett, MD (1970–1982). (Photo provided courtesy of UAB Archives, University of Alabama at Birmingham.)

rare distinction of also holding the title of a Department Chair, leading research pro-grams focused on immunology, bacteriology, and virology in the Department of Micro-biology. In addition to his teaching in rheumatology and the Department of Microbiology (**Fig. 2**), Dr Bennett led efforts to grow faculty and oversaw a substantial growth in research funding at UAB.

The 1970s and 1980s represented a period of historic growth in arthritis research, and Dr Bennett was actively involved in the expansion and promotion of the field of rheumatology. In 1974, the National Arthritis Act was passed,[10] which authorized for-mation of the National Commission on Arthritis and Related Musculoskeletal Diseases. In 1976, the Commission reported to Congress its Arthritis Plan, which called for increased arthritis research and training programs, multipurpose arthritis centers, epidemiologic studies, and data systems in arthritis, a National Arthritis Information Service, and a National Arthritis Advisory Board. Dr Bennett had UAB poised to act at this moment, and in 1977, he became Director of the UAB Multipurpose Arthritis Center, the forerunner of many subsequent NIH-funded program grants led by UAB rheumatologists.

In 1972, while Bennett was the Director of the UAB Division of Rheumatology, the National Institute of Arthritis and Metabolic Diseases (which had been established in 1950) was renamed as the National Institute of Arthritis, Metabolism, and Digestive Diseases.[11] As he transitioned to the role of Chair of the UAB Department of Medicine, Dr Bennett served as President of the American Rheumatism Association (ARA; now

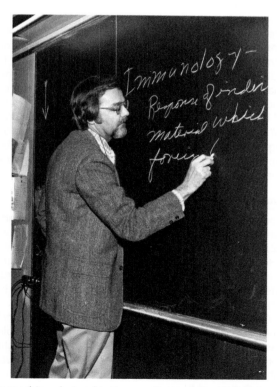

Fig. 2. Dr Bennett teaching during his time as Chair of the UAB Department of Microbi-ology, circa 1976. (Photo provided courtesy of UAB Archives, University of Alabama at Birmingham.)

the American College of Rheumatology). In his 1982 Presidential address,[12] Dr Bennett noted that the US Department of Health and Human Services Secretary Richard S. Schweiker had elevated the NIADDK's programs to division status, creating 5 extramural divisions, including the Division of Arthritis, Musculoskeletal and Skin Diseases. This set the stage for the establishment of the National Institute of Arthritis and Musculoskeletal and Skin Diseases, which occurred in 1986.

During the time of Dr Bennett's national leadership, there were also changes in the professional organizations involved in arthritis and rheumatology. The Arthritis and Rheumatism Foundation (which had been incorporated in 1948) changed its name to the Arthritis Foundation in 1965. Concomitantly, the ARA became the professional section of the Arthritis Foundation. In 1985, 3 years after Bennett had served as ARA President, it separated from the Arthritis Foundation, and in 1988 the ARA changed its name to the American College of Rheumatology.[13]

Dr Bennett was the first holder of the Howard Holley Chair at UAB, named after the founding Director of the UAB Division of Clinical Immunology and Rheumatology (see **Fig. 2**). Bennett served as Editor-in-Chief of *Arthritis & Rheumatism* (now *Arthritis & Rheumatology*) from 1975 to 1980. Importantly, Dr Bennett recruited a number of outstanding rheumatologists and scientists to UAB, including Dr William Koopman (see **Fig. 1**), who succeeded him as Director of the UAB Division of Clinical Immunology and Rheumatology and later as Chair of the UAB Department of Medicine and President of the American College of Rheumatology.

Despite his success in research, arguably Dr Bennett's biggest impact was on advancing the fields of rheumatology and internal medicine. As Chair of the UAB Department of Medicine, he demonstrated remarkable skill at building clinical and research programs, which extended beyond the field of rheumatology. He served as Editor of the *American Journal of Medicine* and on the Board of Governors of the Magnuson Clinical Center at NIH. He was elected President of the Association of American Physicians, President of the Association of Professors of Medicine, and Chair of the American Board of Internal Medicine. In 1986, he was an elected member of the Institute of Medicine (now the National Academy of Medicine). He served as Editor of the *Cecil Textbook of Medicine*, 19th, 20th, and 21st editions. His scientific and clinical background led him to become a staunch advocate for the integration of a didactic curriculum for the sciences into the fabric of clinical training experiences to instill lifelong learning of physicians.[14]

Honors and Awards

Given his many accomplishments in research, program-building, and national leadership, it is not surprising that Dr Bennett received many prestigious awards throughout his career. In 1992, Dr Bennett received an Honorary doctoral Degree from the University of Alabama. He was awarded the Founders Medal from the Southern Society for Clinical Investigation and received the John Phillips Memorial Award for outstanding work in Clinical Medicine from the American College of Physicians based on his lifetime of outstanding innovative impactful work in clinical medicine. He was enrolled into the Alabama Academy of Honor and in 1995, the Arthritis Foundation presented him with their "Humanitarian of the Year" Award. He was the recipient of the Kober Medal from the Association of American Physicians for lifetime achievement based on his enormous impact on the field of Internal Medicine through outstanding leadership and mentorship. He was named a Master of the American College of Physicians (1990) and American College of Rheumatology (1998). The Association of Professors of Medicine bestowed the Robert H. Williams Distinguished Chair of Medicine Award on Dr Bennett in 1994 for his outstanding leadership as the Chair of a Department of

Internal Medicine and contributions to academic internal medicine in the areas of education, research, patient care, and faculty development.

Due in large part to Dr Bennett's leadership, the UAB Division of Clinical Immunology and Rheumatology was named a top-ranked program by *U.S. News & World Report* Best Hospitals when it began its assessments in 1990. For more than 30 years, Rheumatology remained the top-ranked specialty at UAB. Despite offers to lead at the executive level at multiple prestigious medical centers, Dr Bennett remained loyal to UAB. In his Department of Medicine report for 1985, Dr Bennett stated that this was due to his belief that "achieving greatness among Departments of Medicine in the nation is within our grasp."

Dr Bennett was also committed to excellence in medical education and scientific exchange. He held many visiting professorships and invited lectureships at leading academic institutions, not just in the United States but in Europe. He received the Carl Nachman Medal from the German Society of Rheumatology and was elected to the Royal Society of Medicine, London.

Support and Mentorship

Despite his many recognitions, Dr Bennett remained a grounded individual. He took an active interest in the careers of his trainees and was a true friend to his colleagues throughout his career. He helped those around him by facilitating multidisciplinary research to address important scientific questions. On a personal note, Dr Bennett was very supportive of me (Professor Steffen Gay) and my wife Renate when we came to UAB in 1976 from the Max-Planck Institute for Biochemistry in Martinsried Munich/Germany. We worked in the UAB Institute of Dental Research which housed prestigious researchers studying collagens, proteoglycans, glycoproteins, and their immunogenicity. I originally worked with Professor Edward Miller, a prominent collagen researcher. Professor Miller was interested that I was able to produce antibodies to different types of collagen and to study their tissue distribution by immunofluorescence in health and disease, but became interested in autoantibodies to different types of collagen.

At the suggestion of Dr Robert Stroud, a UAB rheumatologist and prominent researcher in complement, we began participating in Rheumatology Grand Rounds which was under the direction of Dr Bennett who was Director of the Division of Rheumatology and Chair of the Department of Microbiology at that time. Dr Bennett and his wife, Nancy Miller Bennett, invited Renate and me to their thanksgiving dinner and our longstanding friendship and collaboration ensued. After Nancy's death, Dr Bennett married Frances Caldwell Bennett in 2002, and Renate and I enjoyed many trips with them through Germany and Switzerland.

Claude became interested in our work with monoclonal antibodies against distinct types of collagens, to study the integrity of basement membranes in tumor invasion. He went with his business colleagues to New York to work with a well-known patent lawyer to develop a patent application for the commercial application of these antibodies. Following the fall of the Berlin Wall, Dr Bennett and Professor Renate Gay created a fellowship Exchange Program between UAB and the Departments of Medicine at the Universities in Leipzig, Germany and the University of Zürich, Switzerland. In tribute to his great efforts to organize this successful program, both the Leipzig University and the University of Zürich gave him a doctoral honoris causa degree.

Dr Bennett was also integral to the success of the Deutsches Rheuma Forschungs Zentrum (DRFZ; German Rheumatology Research Center), a major German rheumatology research center started in Berlin more than 30 years ago. In 1987 Dr Bennett was a member of a group of international experts under the leadership of Professor Fritz Melchers, who was the Director of the Basel Institute for Immunology. This group introduced to the Berlin Senat a new concept for a Research Center in Rheumatology which served as a basis for the DRFZ. Dr Bennett and I were part of the Advisory Committee for the German Rheumatology Research Center. The goal of the DRFZ is to improve health care in patients with rheumatic diseases through research. Drs Bennett and I (Professor Gay) served on the inaugural DRFZ Advisory Committee. Under the scientific leadership of Professor Dr Andreas Radbruch, the DRFZ became an Institute of the famous Leibniz Institute. The Leibniz Association unites 97 independent institutions throughout Germany.

Late Career

On the basis of his substantial success in building programs at UAB and his international reputation as a physician and leader, Bennett was named the fourth President of the University of Alabama at Birmingham in 1993. After 4 years in this role, Dr Bennett was designated by the University Board of Trustees as Distinguished University Professor Emeritus. Of note, Dr Bennett continued to be true to his roots as a physician scientist and remained steadfastly devoted to the development of novel treatments for patients with rheumatic diseases. Thus, he became President and Chief Operating Officer of BioCryst Pharmaceuticals, Inc., where he provided scientific input into drug design and clinical development programs.

Even after his retirement, Dr Bennett, along with his wife Frances, remained as a part of the UAB medical and scientific community, often hosting dinners in their apartment in Birmingham. They were very gracious hosts for dinners in honor of new leaders at UAB and included me (Lou Bridges) and my wife Ginny to help advance the goals of rheumatology within the UAB academic medical center.

In 2020, UAB organized a "Reunion Symposium in Honor of J. Claude Bennett: celebrating 50 Years of Science at UAB". Many of Dr Bennett's friends, colleagues, and collaborators signed on to honor his many accomplishments as a scholar, physician, and leader. Scheduled speakers included Lasker Prize winner Max Cooper, MD; Roy Curtiss, PhD, member of the National Academy of Sciences; and Eric Hunter, PhD, Director of the Center for AIDS Research at Emory University. Unfortunately, this Symposium was scheduled for March 20, 2020, which coincided with the declaration of the COVID-19 pandemic. Despite the last-minute cancellation of the event, Dr Bennett was deeply honored and grateful to the organizers.

After his long and distinguished career, Dr Bennett now resides in Birmingham with his wife Frances, enjoying the company of his many friends and family members. Fittingly, Dr Bennett's family, friends, and colleagues honored him by establishing the J. Claude Bennett Endowed Chair in Rheumatology and Immunology, which will forever acknowledge his long-lasting impact on UAB. Dr Bennett left an indelible mark on the care of patients with rheumatic diseases, on development of new therapeutic approaches based on scientific research, on the careers of his many trainees and colleagues, and on the fields of medicine and rheumatology.

DISCLOSURE

There are no commercial or financial conflicts of interest from either author. There are no relevant funding sources for either author.

REFERENCES

1. The Faculty of Medicine, Harvard University: Edgar Haber. https://fa.hms.harvard. edu/files/hmsofa/files/memorialminute_haber_edgar.pdf. Accessed June 12, 2023.

2. Haber E, Bennett JC. Polarization of fluorescence as a measure of antigen-antibody interaction. Proc Natl Acad Sci U S A 1962;48(11):1935–42.

3. Bennett JC. Genetic Coding for Protein Structure. Annu Rev Biochem 1964;33: 205–34.

4. Archives: The CalTech Archives: Dreyer, William J. https://collections.archives. caltech.edu/agents/people/109. Accessed June 12, 2023.

5. Program in Immunology, UAB Heersink School of Medicine. https://www.uab.edu/ medicine/immunology/bennett.

6. Dreyer WJ, Bennett JC. The molecular basis of antibody formation: a paradox. Proc Natl Acad Sci U S A 1965;54(3):864–9.

7. Sullivan W. Key to antibody origin may be near. New York, NY: The New York Times; 1965. p. 1.

8. Bennett JC. The infectious etiology of rheumatoid arthritis. New considerations. Arthritis Rheum 1978;21(5):531–8.

9. Acton RT, Weinheimer PF, Wolcott M, et al. N-terminal sequences of immunoglobulin heavy and light chains from three species of lower vertebrates. Nature 1970; 228(5275):991–2.

10. Congress.gov. "S.2854 - 93rd Congress (1973-1974): National Arthritis Act." January 4, 1975. https://www.congress.gov/bill/93rd-congress/senate-bill/2854.

11. National Institute of Arthritis, Diabetes, and Digestive and Kidney Diseases (U.S.). Annual report of the national Institute of arthritis, diabetes, and digestive and kidney diseases. Bethesda, MD: Dept. of Health and Human Services, Public Health Service, National Institutes of Health; 1982.

12. Bennett JC. American rheumatology: markings. Presidential address to the American Rheumatism Association, June 1982. Arthritis Rheum 1983 Apr;26(4): 548–52. PMID: 6838678.

13. The History of the American College of Rheumatology Image Library. The Rheumatologist October 19, 2020. Mary Beth Nierengarten. https://www.the-rheumatologist.org/article/the-history-of-the-american-college-of-rheumatology-image-library/#:~:text=In%201985%2C%20the%20ARA%20separated,College %20of%20Rheumatology%20(ACR).

14. Bennett JC. Development of a didactic curriculum in science related to internal medicine. Ann Intern Med 1992;116(12 Pt 2):1088–90.

Edmund Lawrence Dubois (1923–1985)

Daniel J. Wallace, MD, MACR

KEYWORDS

- Lupus • Cedars-Sinai Medical Center • University of Southern California
- Systemic lupus erythematosus • LE cell prep

KEY POINTS

- Edmund Dubois, at the height of his career, had the largest lupus practice in the world.
- He treated more than 2000 patients with the disease between 1950 and 1985.
- He was the first to investigate animal models of lupus and the first to create and establish a basic science laboratory dedicated to understanding the etiopathogenesis of lupus.
- His clinical observations included describing the art of managing lupus with antimalarials, corticosteroids, and immune suppressive agents.
- Dr Dubois' insights laid the groundwork for modern lupus research.

EARLY TRAINING FOR CAREER DEVELOPMENT

Edmund Lawrence Dubois (pronounces Doo-Boyz) was born on June 28, 1923 to a middle-class Jewish family in Newark, New Jersey (**Fig. 1**). He was the only child of a general surgeon father and his mother worked in the office. Ed, as he has been always known, graduated from high school in Newark in 1939. He then attended Johns Hopkins University graduating with a bachelor's degree in 1943. While serving in the Army, he stayed in Baltimore to attend Johns Hopkins Medical School where he completed his internship under A Mc Gehee Harvey, the legendary Chief of Service who was a lupus pioneer in his own right.[1] Ed's tendency to know and train under the best and brightest continued with a residency at the University of Utah under Maxwell Wintrobe (author of the hematology textbook) and at Parkland Hospital in Dallas under Tinsley Harrison (author and editor of Harrison's medical textbook). He also completed an autopsy pathology fellowship at Los Angeles County General Hospital in 1948.

Connecting to Lupus

Ed decided to remain in Southern California and went into private practice in his father's office in July 1950. In 1951, he met and married Nancy Kully, the daughter of

Cedars-Sinai Medical Center, 8750 Wilshire Boulevard, Suite 210, Beverly Hills, CA 90211, USA
E-mail address: Daniel.Wallace@cshs.org

Rheum Dis Clin N Am 50 (2024) 65–71
https://doi.org/10.1016/j.rdc.2023.08.005
0889-857X/24/© 2023 Elsevier Inc. All rights reserved.

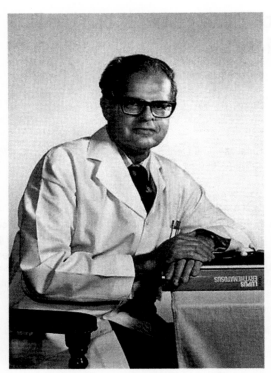

Fig. 1. Giants of rheumatology at Cedars Sinai. Edmund Dubois in 1966. (© Yousuf Karsh.)

Barney Kully who was a community ear, nose, and throat specialist. To keep profes-
sionally busy at the beginning of his career, he volunteered his time at the Los Angeles
County General Hospital. The "General," as it was known, was the largest hospital in
the United States at that time with more than 3000 beds. Dr Paul Starr, then the
Chairman of the Department of Medicine at the General, asked him to start a new clinic
consisting of eight patients who had a recently diagnosed disorder characterized by
the presence of a newly described laboratory test known as the lupus erythematosus
(LE) cell prep. The LE prep was the first specific test for lupus and antedated the antinuclear antibody (ANA) by 9 years. The test was first performed by Malcolm Hargraves
at the Mayo Clinic in 1948. The LE prep was very complex to perform consistently and
accurately. Eventually, it became the prototype of the anti-histone antibody test; the
test became obsolete quickly because it could never be mechanized or made practical and required specialized beaded tubes to perform.[2] The word spread quickly
about Ed's availability and clinical skills and competence. Within 10 years, Ed had
amassed the largest lupus practice in the world caring for 500 patients at the Tuesday
morning Lupus Clinic at the General and another 500 in his Beverly Hills private practice office. For the purposes of reference, UCLA graduated its first medical school
class in 1955, and Cedars of Lebanon and Mount Sinai Hospitals merged to form
Cedars-Sinai Medical Center in 1961.

By the mid-1980s, over half of the rheumatologists in Southern California could say
confidently that Ed Dubois had taught them nearly everything they would need to
know about lupus. His initial publications seemed in the *Journal of the American*

Medical Association, Archives of Internal Medicine,[2,3] and the *American Journal of Medicine.*[3–6] These pivotal publications described autoimmune hemolytic anemia as a manifestation of systemic lupus erythematosus (SLE), showed that steroids could ameliorate the disease, and described the general clinical and laboratory features of patients who had positive LE cell preps.

Practicing at Cedars of Lebanon and the University of Southern California

In 1954, he joined what may have been one of the most accomplished and successful elite internal medicine private practices in the country, which included Myron Prinzmetal (known for Prinzmetal' s angina) and Eliot Corday (coinventor of the Holter monitor with Norman J Holter).[7,8] His father-in-law became the medical director of Metro Goldwyn Mayer (MGM) under Louis B Mayer, and Ed included Judy Garland, Zsa Zsa Gabor, and other luminaries as his patients. He bought his first house from Ronald Colman.

Accomplishments

As the General became more closely affiliated with the University of Southern California (USC), university resources allowed the establishment of a lupus research laboratory. Ed Dubois' keen clinical instincts and his demands for perfection among those who worked with him permitted him to publish seminal works which established him among the very first to propose insights that we now take for granted. These "firsts" include the following contributions from 1954 to 1978.[9–30]

Use of nitrogen mustard for serious SLE (1954)
Use of quinacrine for cutaneous and mild lupus (1954)
High-dose steroid protocol for managing central nervous system disease (1956)
Hydralazine induction of LE cells (1957)
First description of avascular necrosis with Lewis Cozen (author of 8 textbooks in orthopedic surgery) (1960)
First description of steroid-induced peptic ulcers (1960)
First description of gangrene from lupus vasculitis (1962)
Cutaneous disease and light sensitivity in lupus (1963)
Establishment of the first New Zealand Brown/New Zealnad White (NZB/NZW) mouse research laboratory (1963)
Mechanisms of antimalarial retinal toxicity (1963)
Detailed and incredible analysis of an accrued series of 520 lupus patients (1964)
LE cells that occur after oral contraceptives (1967)
Use of cyclophosphamide for SLE (1967)
First large series of procainamide induced lupus (1968)
Absence of erosions in lupus synovitis (1970)
Phenothiazine-induced lupus large series (1972)
Interstitial lung disease in lupus (1974)
First analysis of causes of death among 212 patients (1974)—he attended many of their funerals.
Human leukocyte antiben (HLA) typing of lupus patients (1974)
Ibuprofen for SLE (1975)
Review of septic arthritis in lupus (1975)
Familial lupus (1978)

Legacy

In 1966, Ed wrote the first edition of his monograph, *Lupus Erythematosus: A review of the current status of discoid and systemic lupus erythematosus and their variants* published by Mc Graw Hill. Dedicated "to the patients who we have learned," this remarkable largely single-authored textbook was enormously successful and is now in its 10th edition. More than any other publication, this textbook has shaped how rheumatologists approach and treat the disease. He created this textbook and, at the same time, was able to author numerous peer-reviewed articles. In addition to his academic work, he founded The American Lupus Society to promote patient involvement and advocacy.

Ed Dubois the Person

Ed Dubois was a tireless workaholic. He would rise at 5 AM and write for an hour or two before going to work. A humanist of the first order, half of his time was spent providing free medical care. He was exacting and did not suffer fools easily. Although he seemed to be a man of few words, his gentle kind-heartedness was always evident. Ed's probing intellect was apparent within moments of meeting him, and he was always relaxed, modest, and approachable. Ed could be a wonderful teacher when meeting with a student physician with an inquiring mind and a capacity to work hard. He was never snobbish and conceited and felt more at home seeing indigent patients than hobnobbing with Hollywood luminaries.

On a personal level, I remember that Ed would never fail to give his fellows a good meal during the American Rheumatology Association (ARA) (precursor of the American College of Rheumatology [ACR]) meetings. I also remember him introducing me to an elegant Eric Bywaters in the late 1970s, resplendent in his Edwardian tweed suit and Sherlock Holmes hat reviewing my poster. More than anything else, Ed Dubois was a private man devoted to his family. He was happily married, had four children, all of whom have had successful careers. His first grandchild was born shortly before he passed away. An expert yachtsman who relaxed best on his boat (when he was terminally ill, he bought a new boat that he named "Dubious"). His other consuming passion was photography. Able to be privately tutored by the likes of Ansel Adams, his office was filled with creative and wonderful pictures showing his love for life.

The Los Angeles Medical Environment During Ed's Life in 1950 to 1977

The clinical practice of medicine in West Los Angeles in 1950 was arduous. It included going to several small hospitals a day, reading x-rays that were ordered, making lots of house calls, and charging about $5 a visit. Ed's practice model was innovative for its time and has not been duplicated since. He scheduled six patients each at 9 AM, 10:30 AM, 1 PM, and 2:30 PM. On clinic days as the patients arrived, a nurse took their vital signs and drew their blood as Dr Dubois circulated among them. For 20 years and while chain smoking, Marlene Rogers drew LE cell preps on all of them at every visit and performed the testing on the spot. A strong bond developed between, for example, the 10:30 Thursday group, and the patients became friends and often went for lunch or coffee together. Trying to get into a specific group sometimes led to turf-related altercations. Mavis Cox (his assistant) lived on a farm in El Monte, California, and raised chickens, goats, and rabbits while maintaining his lupus library and coordinating his General Hospital lupus clinic.

The "Questionable" Division of Rheumatology

Ed developed lifelong friendships with his colleagues at the USC and Cedars of Lebanon (later Cedars-Sinai Medical Center). At USC, these included George Friou (who was the first to describe the fluorescent antinuclear antibody and anti-double stranded deoxynucleic acid [dsDNA] tests),[31,32] Sam Rappaport and Don Feinstein (who were among the first to describe the lupus anticoagulant),[33] and Frank Quismorio, who took over his clinic on Ed's retirement.

At Cedars-Sinai Medical Center, he was close with Jim Klinenberg (past ACR president who was the first to describe the clinical effects of allopurinol) and Marshal Fichman (who saw hundreds of his nephritis patients). Before Cedars-Sinai offering rheumatology fellowships (originally in combination with UCLA) in 1971, Ed played a significant role in molding what had been a division of questionable value. The scene around that part of Los Angeles was quite remarkable and brings back many memories of my training. The Division of Rheumatology at that time was replete with a "Damon Runyon"-esque atmosphere. In the 1960s, the head of the Gold clinic was a malpractice attorney and rheumatologist who sued his Cedars colleagues. It also included a connected Hollywood rheumatologist who hired residents to go to movie star houses each night between 9 and 11 PM to inject them with pentobarbital (Nembutal) so they could sleep. When I was a fellow this attending denounced HLA-B27 as a hoax and fake news due to antipathy toward one of the original UCLA investigators. When I tried to dispute this once on teaching rounds, he loudly walked out of the patient's room in a huff.

Final Illness

Although still a youthful 54 years of age in 1977, Ed complained of knee and low back pain which turned out to be a compression fracture from multiple myeloma. He privately confided to me that excessive exposure to radiation during his training in various research laboratories was responsible. He lived for another 8 years after getting experimental treatment from Dr Robert Kyle at the Mayo Clinic. He saw a full schedule of patients before succumbing to pneumonia 2 weeks before passing away in February 1985.

In 1977, while a first-year rheumatology fellow for the then combined Cedars-Sinai/UCLA Rheumatology Fellowship program (they are separated and distinct, currently), I was called into Jim Klinenberg's office. Jim was the director of the Department of Internal Medicine at Cedars-Sinai and wanted to know if could see Ed's new patients with him in his office 1 day a week in view of Ed's immobility. This evolved to an amazing friendship, and Ed ultimately invited me to evaluate his entire cohort, to take over his practice, and ultimately to edit the third edition of his textbook with him.[34–36] We later recruited Bevra Hahn to assist in the endeavor. Being able to spend time and have Ed mentor me was one of the highlights of my professional career, and the observation of such an individual who was so tirelessly dedicated to his patients is a lesson that I will never forget. Are those lessons available today?

CLINICS CARE POINTS

- Edmund Dubois advanced the field of systemic lupus as a result of his work.
- He established the largest cohort of lupus patients published at the time and characterized their clinical and laboratory aspects, prognosis and treatment.
- He will be remembered for his clinical insights and his legacy includes writing the first 3 editions of the definitive lupus textbook named in his honoe.

DISCLOSURE

Dr D.J. Wallace has no conflicts of interest.

REFERENCES

1. Harvey AM, Howard JE, Winkenwerder WL, et al. Observations on the Effect of Adrenocorticotrophic Hormone (ACTH) on Disseminated Lupus Erythematosus, Drug Hypersensitivity Reactions, and Chronic Bronchial Asthma. Trans Am Clin Climatol Assoc 1949;61:221–8. PMID: 21407721 F.
2. Hargraves M, Richmond H, Morton R. Presentation of two bone marrow components, the tart cell and the LE cell. Mayo Clin Proc 1948;27:25–8.
3. Dubois EL. Simplified method for the L. E. cell test; results of a three-year study of seven hundred tests in many disease states. Arch Intern Med 1953;92(2):168–84. PMID: 13079337 No abstract available.
4. Dubois EL. The effect of the L. E. cell test on the clinical picture of systemic lupus erythematosus. Ann Intern Med 1953;38(6):1265–94. PMID: 13065975 No abstract available.
5. Dubois EL, Commons RR, Starr P, et al. Corticotropin and cortisone treatment for systemic lupus erythematosus. Am Med Assoc 1952;149(11):995–1002. PMID: 14938089 No abstract available. Share.
6. Dubois EL. Acquired hemolytic anemias the presenting syndrome of lupus erythematosus disseminatus. Am J Med 1952;12(2):197–204.
7. Prinzmetal M, Kennamer R, Merliss R, et al. Angina pectoris. I. A variant form of angina pectoris. Preliminary report. Am J Med 1959;27:375–88.
8. Delmar B. The history of Clinical Holter Monitoring. Ann Noninvasive Electrocardiol 2005;10(2):226–30.
9. Dubois ELAMA. Nitrogen mustard in treatment of systemic lupus erythematosus. Arch Intern Med 1954;93(5):667–72.
10. Dubois EL. AMA. Quinacrine (atabrine) in treatment of systemic and discoid lupus erythematosus. Arch Intern Med 1954;94(1):131–41. PMID: 13170849 No abstract available.
11. Dubois EL. Prednisone and prednisolone in the treatment of systemic lupus erythematous. J Am Med Assoc 1956;161(5):427–33. PMID: 13318931 No abstract available.
12. Dubois EL, Katz YJ, Freeman V, et al. Chronic toxicity studies of hydralazine (apresoline) in dogs with particular reference to the production of the hydralazine syndrome. Lab Clin Med 1957;50(1):119–26. PMID: 13439273 No abstract available.
13. Dubois EL, Cozen L. Avascular (aseptic) bone necrosis associated with systemic lupus erythematosus. JAMA 1960;174:966–71. PMID: 13724595 No abstract available.
14. Dubois EL, Bulgrin JG, Jacobson G. The corticosteroid-induced peptic ulcer. Am J Gastroenterol 1960;33:435–53. PMID: 13818309 No abstract available.
15. Dubois EL, Arterberry JD. Gangrene as a manifestation of systemic lupus erythematosus. JAMA 1962;181:366–74. PMID: 13888052 No abstract available.
16. Tuffanelli DL, Dubois EL. Cutaneous manifestations of systemic lupus erythematosus. Arch Dermatol 1964 Oct;90:377–86. PMID: 14184481.
17. Dubois EL, Horowitz RE, Demopoulos HB, et al. NZB/NZW mice as a model of systemic lupus erythematosus. JAMA 1966;195(4):285–9. PMID: 4159181 No abstract available.
18. Shearer RV, Dubois EL. Ocular changes induced by long-term hydroxychloroquine (plaquenil) therapy. Am J Ophthalmol 1967;64(2):245–52. PMID: 6036279 No abstract available.

19. Dubois EL, Tuffanelli DL. Clinical manifestations of systemic lupus erythematosus. computer analysis of 520 cases. JAMA 1964;190:104–11. PMID: 14184513 No abstract available.
20. DuBois EL, Strain L, Ehn M, et al. cells after oral contraceptives. Lancet 1968; 2(7569):679. PMID: 4175508 No abstract available.
21. Horowitz RE, Dubois EL, Weiner J, et al. Cyclophosphamide treatment of mouse systemic lupus erythematosus. Lab Invest 1969;21(3):199–206. PMID: 4185855 No abstract available.
22. Molina J, Dubois EL, Bilitch M, et al. Procainamide-induced serologic changes in asymptomatic patients. Arthritis Rheum 1969;12(6):608–14. PMID: 4188607 No abstract available.
23. Dubois EL, Tallman E, Wonka RA. Chlorpromazine-induced systemic lupus erythematosus: case report and review of the literature. JAMA 1972;221(6):595–6. PMID: 4114624 No abstract available.
24. Dubois EL, Friou GJ, Chandor S. Rheumatoid nodules and rheumatoid granulomas in systemic lupus erythematosus. JAMA 1972;220(4):515–8. PMID: 5067126 No abstract available.
25. Eisenberg H, Dubois EL, Sherwin RP, et al. Diffuse interstitial lung disease in systemic lupus erythematosus. Ann Intern Med 1973;79(1):37–45. PMID.
26. Dubois EL, Wierzchowiecki M, Cox MB, et al. Duration and death in systemic lupus erythematosus. An analysis of 249 cases. JAMA 1974;227(12):1399–402. PMID: 4406022 No abstract available.
27. Nies KM, Brown JC, Dubois EL, et al. Histocompatibility (HL-A) antigens and lymphocytotoxic antibodies in systemic lupus erythematosus (SLE). Arthritis Rheum 1974;17(4):397–402. PMID: 4852277 No abstract available.
28. Dubois EL. Letter: Ibuprofen for systemic lupus erythematosus. N Engl J Med 1975;293(15):779. No abstract available.
29. Quismorio FP, Dubois EL. Septic arthritis in systemic lupus erythematosus. J Rheumatol 1975;2(1):73–82. PMID: 1185738.
30. Buckman KJ, Moore SK, Ebbin AJ, et al. Familial systemic lupus erythematosus. Arch Intern Med 1978;138(11):1674–6. PMID: 718317.
31. Friou GJ, Finch SC, Detre KD. Interaction of nuclei and globulin from lupus erythematosis serum demonstrated with fluorescent antibody. J Immunol 1958;80(4): 324–9. PMID: 13539376.
32. Friou GJ. The early days of the antinuclear antibody story: where and how did it all start. Ann Med Intenr (Paris) 1993;144:154–6.
33. Feinstein DI, Rapaport SI. Acquired inhibitors of blood coagulation. Prog Hemost Thromb 1972;1:75–195.
34. Wallace DJ, Podell TE, Weiner JM, et al. Lupus nephritis. Experience with 230 patients in a private practice from 1950 to 1980. Am J Med 1982;72(2):209–20.
35. Wallace DJ, Podell T, Weiner J, et al. Systemic lupus erythematosus–survival patterns. Experience with 609 patients. JAMA 1981;245(9):934–8.
36. Dubois' lupus erythematosus, 3rd edition, Lea & Febiger, Philadelphia, PA, Edited by Edmund L, Dubois and Daniel J W,1985.

Lessons from Carl M. Pearson 1919 – 1981

James S. Louie, MD, MACR

KEYWORDS

• University of California in Los Angeles • HLA-B27 • UCLA • Myositis

Carl M. Pearson was an energetic and exceptional physician–scholar-leader who founded, established, and broadened the Divisions of Rheumatology at University of California in Los Angeles (UCLA) beginning in 1956. As his education and insatiable scientific curiosity enabled him to pursue the science of genetic and inflammatory muscle diseases, his remarkable insight to pleasantly engage, collaborate, recruit, and enable the diverse talents of many throughout the world generated signal investigations in diverse diseases, which enhanced the commitment and service of all who trained within the UCLA Divisions of Rheumatology.

Dr Pearson was born in Seattle, Washington, November 9, 1919. After receiving his BA degree at UCLA and MD from Boston University, he trained in pathology at the Boston City and Massachusetts General where he investigated animal models of muscle diseases[1–3] and coauthored *Diseases of Muscle: A Study in Pathology* with Raymond Adams and D. Denny Brown. His studies to induce myositis by injecting muscle saturated with the heat-killed tubercle bacillus, an emulsifier, and mineral oil (Freund's adjuvant) enabled his report that polyarthritis occurred with Freund's adjuvant alone in certain strains of rat and mice. This model of adjuvant arthritis allowed the next generation of studies to assess therapies for autoimmune diseases. Carl was always using control!

Clinically, Dr Pearson also trained in Internal Medicine before his service in Japan during the Korean conflict and in Rheumatology at the Lahey Clinic before his selection to become Chief of Rheumatology at UCLA in Westwood. As the initial Chief of Rheumatology, Dr Pearson secured funding for both the Division of Rheumatology offices and laboratories at the Rehabilitation Center and for the Jerry Lewis Neuromuscular Disease Center. He also served on the Executive committees for the Arthritis Rheumatism Association (now American College of Rheumatology), Arthritis Foundation, and Muscular Dystrophy Associations.

To establish the Division with a broad investigative commitment, Carl recruited James Peter, MD, PhD, who studied oxidative phosphorylation with Paul Boyer, eventual Nobel winner[4,5]; James Klinenberg who studied oxypurines and the xanthine oxidase therapies for gout with J Seegmiller at the NIH[6,7]; and Eugene Barnett who

Rheumatology and Arthritis, UCLA, Los Angeles, CA, USA
E-mail address: jlouie@mednet.ucla.edu

Rheum Dis Clin N Am 50 (2024) 73–77
https://doi.org/10.1016/j.rdc.2023.08.006
0889-857X/24/© 2023 Published by Elsevier Inc.

rheumatic.theclinics.com

described the testing and therapies for autosensitivity diseases including systemic lupus with John Vaughan at University of Rochester.[8–10]

When Dr Pearson and these investigators secured a United State Public Health Service grant to investigate the pharmacology and toxicology of therapeutic mechanisms of rheumatic disease, Carl recruited investigational and clinical pharmacologists, Michael Whitehouse,[11] Yi-Han Chang,[12] Nirmal Kar,[13,14] and Harold Paulus,[15–17] who spearheaded the immunologic and clinical studies from the lymphocytes removed from the thoracic duct.

Dr Pearson energized the Rheumatology program by enabling diverse collaborations in investigations, teaching, and apt clinical care. His first Fellows included Randall Parker who constructed a simplified synovial biopsy instrument called the Parker-Pearson needle,[18] which was subsequently validated by his co-Fellow, Ralph Schumacher, who became the quintessential physician-scientist at the University of Pennsylvania VA in Philadelphia[19–21]; Anthony Cracchiolo, orthopedic surgeon, who described immune responses and hydrolases in arthritis synovium[22–24] before establishing the UCLA unit for Orthopedic Foot and Ankle clinic; Sherman Mellinkoff, gastroenterologist, who described that high-protein diets decreased adjuvant arthritis[25] before serving as Dean of UCLA; and Anthony Verity, neuropathologist.[26,27] Indeed, Carl Pearson's commitment to innovative clinical care of diverse muscle diseases prompted James Peter and Anthony Bohan to describe the clinical criteria for polymyositis,[28–30] and Stuart Novack, David Yu, and Peng Fan to be among the first to study immunosuppressive drugs for Wegener's granulomatosis, and corticosteroids therapeutic effects on immune mechanisms.[31–35]

In addition, Dr Pearson selected new Chiefs with collaborative skills to lead at the affiliated UCLA Medical Center and thus expanded the capabilities for the scientific and clinical training of Fellows and postdoctoral investigators. These UCLA Fellows shared their diverse interests and skills to lead Rheumatology investigations and clinical care throughout the world. James Klinenberg began Rheumatology Fellowships at Cedars Sinai Medical Center before becoming Chief of Medicine. Rodney Bluestone, the prototypic English investigator-clinician with his articulate, prompting, and decisive teaching skills, developed the collaborative Fellowship program at the Wadsworth (now West Los Angeles) VA hospital where he facilitated Lee Schlosstein's and Paul Terasaki's description of HLA-B27 in the spondyloarthropathies.[36–38] Although Seymour White was collaborating with UCLA Dermatology to describe the first association of a medical disease (psoriasis) with HLA genes, Rodney Bluestone assigned Lee to search for an HLA genetic association with gout. Lee collected more than 60 patients with gout from all of the affiliated UCLA divisions when he discovered that 9 of the 10 controls with ankylosing spondylitis were HLA-B27 positive. I remember helping Lee Schlosstein rehearse his presentation for the annual rheumatology meeting in New York when his nervousness made him lose his voice and he had to drink a glass of water at the podium before he could continue! At Mama Leone's restaurant, Lee confided to me that he did not enjoy presenting and would move away from academic sites. He remained in control and became one of the first clinical Rheumatologist in Anchorage, Alaska.

Dr Pearson selected the studious Richard Weisbart to head the Rheumatology Division at the Sepulveda VA where Richard continued his investigations of molecular mechanisms that affected autoimmune and cancer diseases and trained several Fellows into academic, biotechnologic and clinical leadership positions, including Andrew Wong, the current Chief, and Deborah Zack. Carl counseled me to chair the Division of Rheumatology at LAC Harbor UCLA Medical Center with Ken Nies and Michael Liebling. We reported on the outcomes of systemic lupus and infectious diseases and were among the first to facilitate earlier diagnoses of Lyme, tuberculosis, and gonococcal diseases by polymerase chain reaction. Our students and Fellows found leadership roles at the West Los Angeles VA, Martin Luther King, Mayo Clinic, and PLA Hospitals in China.

As the Divisions of Rheumatology grew, Carl reached out to recruit and enable investigators and postdoctoral students from throughout the world—particularly Australia, England, Canada, China, Hong Kong, Singapore, Japan, and United Arab Emirates. Following work with Henri Kunkel, David Yu trained research fellows now leading at the Massachusetts General, Sun Yat-sen University in Guangzhou and the PLA hospital in Beijing.[31–35]

For most of us who trained as Fellows and postdocs, Carl advised and facilitated our academic and personal pursuits as we progressed in our careers. His academic life to ask Why with focused investigations and How to facilitate the collaborative interests and expertise of others served as exemplary lessons for us all. Indeed, Dr Pearson's successor as Chief, Dr Bevra Hahn, continued his legacy, recruiting more than 25 research and clinical investigators for basic and clinical investigations in systemic sclerosis, gout, vasculitis while continuing her investigations in systemic lupus erythematosus, and her commitment for mentoring and teaching. Dr Christina Charles-Schoeman, the current Chief, has continued Carl's legacy, spearheading investigations of lipoproteins inducing inflammatory changes in joints and, interestingly, inflammatory muscle diseases while continuing one of the largest Fellowship program in the United States.

Most of us had the privilege to sit with Carl and thank him for his academic and often personal counsel and support in his final months as he succumbed from his cancer. We marveled at how his dedication to scientific, clinical, and innovative therapeutics and his personal outreach both to colleagues and to patients taught us to achieve as teachers of Rheumatology and knowledgeable clinicians at sites throughout the world.

REFERENCES

1. Wood FD. Pearson CM Protection of rats against adjuvant arthritis by bacterial lipopolysaccharides. Science 1962;137(3529):544–5.

2. Pearson CM, Wood FD. Studies of arthritis and other lesions induced in rats by the injection of mycobacterial adjuvant. VII. Pathologic details of the arthritis and spondylitis. Am J Pathol 1963;42(1):73–95.

3. Pearson CM. Wood FD Passive Transfer of Adjuvant Arthritis by Lymph Node or Spleen Cells. J Exp Med 1964;120(4):547–60.

4. Peter JB, Boyer PD. The formation of bound phosphohistidine from adenosine triphosphate-P32 in mitochondria. J Biol Chem 1963;238:1180–2.

5. Peter JB, Hultquist DE, Deluca M, et al. Bound phosphohistidine as an intermediate in a phosphorylation reaction of oxidative phosphorylation catalyzed by mitochondrial extracts. J Biol Chem 1963;238:1182–4.

6. Klinenberg JR, Bluestone R, Schlosstein L, et al. How is it regulated and how can it be modified? Ann Intern Med 1973;78(1):99–111.

7. Kippen I, Whitehouse MW, Klinenberg JR. Pharmacology of uricosuric drugs. Ann Rheum Dis 1974;33(4):391–6.

8. Bickel YB, Barnett EV, Pearson CM. Immunofluorescent patterns and specificity of human antinuclear antibodies. Clin Exp Immunol 1968;3(7):641–56.

9. Drinkard JP, Stanley TM, Dornfeld L, et al. Azathioprine and prednisone in the treatment of adults with lupus nephritis. Clinical, histological, and immunological changes with therapy. Medicine (Baltim) 1970;49(5):411–32.

10. Abe C, Chia D, Barnett EV, et al. Effects of water-soluble adjuvant (WSA) on New Zealand (NZB X NZW) F1 hybrid mice. Clin Immunol Immunopathol 1977;8(1): 17–27.

11. Whitehouse DJ, Whitehouse MW, Pearson CM. Passive transfer of adjuvant-arthritis and allergic encephalomyelitis in rats using thoracic duct drainage. Nature 1969;224:1322.

12. Chang YH, Pearson CM, Abe C. Adjuvant polyarthritis IV. Induction by a synthetic adjuvant: immunologi, histopathologic and other studies. Arthritis Rheum 1980; 23:62–71.

13. Kar NC, Pearson CM. Glyoxalase enzyme system in human muscular dystrophy. Clin Chim Acta 1975;65(1):153–5.

14. Kar NC, Pearson CM. Acid, neutral and alkaline cathepsins in normal and diseased human muscle. Enzyme 1972;3(4):188–96.

15. Pearson CM, Paulus HE. Machleder HI The role of the lymphocyte and its products in the propagation of joint disease. Ann N Y Acad Sci 1975;256:150–68.

16. Paulus HE, Machleder H, Bangert R, et al. A case report: thoracic duct lymphocyte drainage in rheumatoid arthritis. Clin Immunol Immunopathol 1973;1(2): 173–81.

17. Emori HW, Paulus H, Bluestone R, et al. Indomethacin serum concentrations in man. Effects of dosage, food, and antacid. Ann Rheum Dis 1976;35(4):333–8.

18. Parker RH, Pearson CM. A simplified synovial biopsy needle. Arthritis Rheum 1963;6:172–6.

19. Schumacher HR Jr, Kulka JP. Needle biopsy of the synovial membrane–experience with the Parker-Pearson technic. N Engl J Med 1972;286(8):416–9.

20. Schumacher HR, Szekely IE, Park SA, et al. Acute leukemic cells. Qualitative and quantitative electron microscopy. Am J Pathol 1973;73:27–46.

21. Zhang LY, Ogdie AR, Schumacher HR. Light and electron microscopic features of synovium in patients with psoriatic arthritis. Ultrastruct Pathol 2012;36:207–18.

22. Kar NC, Cracchiolo A 3rd, Mirra J, et al. Acid, neutral, and alkaline hydrolases in arthritic synovium. Am J Clin Pathol 1976;65(2):220–8.

23. Bluestone R, Cracchiolo A 3rd, Goldberg LS, et al. Catabolism and synovial transport of rheumatoid factor. Ann Rheum Dis 1970;29(1):47–55.

24. Pearson CM, Amstutz HC, Bluestone R, et al. UCLA Conference. Diagnosis and treatment of erosive rheumatoid arthritis and other forms of joint destruction. Ann Intern Med 1975;82(2):241–56.

25. Mellinkoff SM, Pearson CM, Wood FD, et al. Studies of polyarthritis induced in rats by injection of mycobacterial adjuvant. VI. Effects of dietary alterations. Am J Clin Nutr 1962;10:398–402.

26. Cancilla PA, Kalyanaraman K, Verity MA, et al. Familial myopathy with probable lysis of myofibrils in type I fibers. Neurology 1971;21(6):579–85.

27. Verity MA, Toop J, McAdam LP, et al. Histochemical and electron microscopic observations. Am J Clin Pathol 1978;69(4):446–51.

28. Bohan A, Peter JB. Polymyositis and dermatomyositis (second of two parts). N Engl J Med 1975;292(8):403–7.

29. Bohan A, Peter JB. Polymyositis and dermatomyositis (first of two parts). N Engl J Med 1975;292(7):344–7.

30. Bohan A, Peter JB, Bowman RL, et al. Computer-assisted analysis of 153 patients with polymyositis and dermatomyositis. Medicine (Baltim) 1977;56(4):255–86.

31. Novack SN, Pearson CM. Cyclophosphamide therapy in Wegener's Granuloma-tosis. New Engl J Medicine 1971;284(17):938–42.
32. Yu DT, Clements PJ, Pearson CM. Effect of corticosteroids on exercise-induced lymphocytosis. Clin Exp Immunol 1977;28(2):326–31.
33. Fan PT, Yu DT, Pearson CM, et al. Human monocyte-lymphocyte interaction: a new technique. J Immunol 1977;119(1):156–61.
34. Yu DT, Choo SY, Schaack T. Molecular mimicry in HLA-B27-related arthritis. Ann Intern Med 1989;111(7):581–91.
35. Zhu J, Yu DT. Matrix metalloproteinase expression in the spondyloarthropathies. Curr Opin Rheumatol 2006;18(4):364–8.
36. White SH, Newcomer VD, Mickey MR, et al. Disturubance of HL-A antigen fre-quency in Psoriasis. N Engl J Med 1972;287:740–3.
37. Schlosstein L, Terasaki PI, Bluestone R, et al. High association of an HL-A anti-gen, W27, with ankylosing spondylitis. N Engl J Med 1973;288(14):704–6.
38. Bluestone R, Pearson CM. Ankylosing spondylitis and Reiter's syndrome: their interrelationship and association with HLA B27. Adv Intern Med 1977;22:1–19.

Walter Bauer, Marian Wilkins Ropes, and the Massachusetts General Hospital

Anthony M. Reginato, PhD, MD[a,b], Michelle A. Petri, MD, MPH[c],
Jonathan Kay, MD[d,*]

KEYWORDS

- Walter Bauer • Marian Wilkins Ropes • Massachusetts General Hospital
- Rheumatology • History • Synovial fluid • Rheumatoid arthritis
- Systemic lupus erythematosus

KEY POINTS

- Walter Bauer advocated for integrating medical research with patient care and teaching in the academic medical center to advance medical knowledge.
- Bauer approached the study of rheumatic diseases both by careful clinical observation and description and by bringing basic scientists and clinicians together to study the anatomy and physiology of connective tissue in the laboratory.
- Marian Wilkins Ropes was a pioneering woman in medicine and was the first female rheumatologist in the United States to have a productive academic career, both in research and clinical care.
- Bauer and Ropes collaborated to study the physical and chemical properties of synovial fluid and reported their comprehensive analysis of pathological findings in synovial fluid from various joint diseases in a classic book published in 1953.

INTRODUCTION AND OVERVIEW

Until the early 20th century, patients with arthritis had been cared for by orthopedic surgeons. At a European meeting of medical hydrology in 1925, Jan van Bremen organized several European physicians to collaborate in the study and treatment of rheumatic diseases, which resulted in the formation of La Ligue Internationale Contre le

Funding: None.
[a] Division of Rheumatology, Department of Medicine, Rhode Island Hospital, Warren Alpert Medical School of Brown University, Providence, RI 02903, USA; [b] Department of Dermatology, Rhode Island Hospital, Warren Alpert Medical School of Brown University, Providence, RI 02903, USA; [c] Division of Rheumatology, Department of Medicine, Johns Hopkins School of Medicine, Baltimore, MD 21287, USA; [d] Division of Rheumatology, Department of Medicine, UMass Chan Medical School, UMass Memorial Medical Center, Worcester, MA 01605, USA
* Corresponding author. 119 Belmont Street, Worcester, MA 01605.
E-mail address: jonathan.kay@umassmemorial.org

Rheum Dis Clin N Am 50 (2024) 79–92
https://doi.org/10.1016/j.rdc.2023.09.001
0889-857X/24/© 2023 Elsevier Inc. All rights reserved.

rheumatic.theclinics.com

Rhumatisme in 1928.[1,2] That same year, the American Committee for the Control of Rheumatism was established with 14 members, including Ralph Pemberton of Philadelphia as its chair.[3] Its purpose was "to stimulate professional and lay interest in arthritis, research and education, the development of a nomenclature and to publicize therapeutic measures of proven value."

In 1926 at the Mayo Clinic in Rochester, Minnesota, Philip S. Hench established the first American academic division devoted to the study and treatment of patients with arthritis and as a resource to educating residents and fellows in this discipline.[3] Three years later, in 1929, similar academic units were established at the Massachusetts General Hospital (MGH) and Harvard Medical School in Boston by Walter Bauer and at Columbia-Presbyterian Hospital in New York City by Ralph H. Boots. Between 1932 and 1937, additional such academic units were founded at the New York University School of Medicine in New York City by Currier McEwen, at the University of Michigan Medical School in Ann Arbor by Richard H. Freyberg, and at the Hospital of the University of Pennsylvania in Philadelphia by Bernard Comroe.[4]

Because Walter Bauer believed that pathology would provide the appropriate background for detailed observation and description of rheumatic diseases, he brought basic scientists into the hospital to work side-by-side with clinicians in the MGH Arthritis Unit. K. Frank Austen pointed out that Bauer "emphasized the importance of acknowledging what one did not know when providing patient care, specifically to patients with inflammatory arthritis."[5] This approach resulted in definitive descriptions of the clinical presentation and pathology of rheumatoid arthritis and other rheumatic diseases. Bauer was joined by Marian Wilkins Ropes, one of the first female rheumatologists in the nation. Both Bauer and Ropes provided leadership to the members of the MGH Arthritis Unit in combining clinical observation and clinical care with basic science laboratory investigations to further the understanding of the rheumatic diseases. This article discusses key contributions of these "*giants in rheumatology*" to illustrate their contributions to clinical medicine, scientific research, and leadership of American rheumatology.

WALTER BAUER (1898–1963)

Walter Bauer was born in Crystal Falls, Michigan, in 1898[6–9] (**Fig. 1**) .He received his bachelor of science from the University of Michigan in 1920 and his medical degree from the University of Michigan Medical School in 1922.[9] After graduation, Bauer was an intern in medicine at the Long Island College Hospital in Brooklyn, New York.[6] Discouraged by the number of patients he observed for whom he could provide only symptomatic care,[8] he moved to Boston in 1923, where he spent a year working with Joseph C. Aub at Harvard Medical School studying the secretions of the adrenal gland.[9] The following year, he was appointed as a resident physician at the MGH.[8,9] In 1927, he traveled to England, where he spent a year studying liver metabolism as a National Research Council Fellow in the Department of Biochemistry and Pharmacology at the National Institute for Medical Research in London, under the guidance of the Nobel laureate and physiologist Sir Henry Hallett Dale.

Upon returning to the MGH, Bauer was appointed as an assistant in medicine and worked with Aub and Fuller Albright as a member of the metabolic research team on Ward 4.[8,10,11] In 1929, he was invited to organize a new research program in diseases of bones, joints, and connective tissue and founded the Robert W. Lovett Memorial Unit for the Study of Crippling Diseases, which he directed from 1929 to 1958.[8,10,11] During that time, he advanced through the clinical ranks at the MGH, from assistant physician to associate physician, and finally to physician.[10] At Harvard Medical

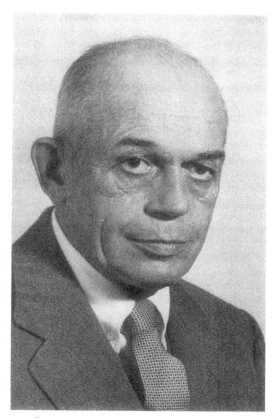

Fig. 1. Dr. Walter Bauer.[7] (*From* Bywaters EGL. Walter Bauer, 1898-1963. Ann Rheum Dis 1964;23(2):170-171.)

School, he was appointed as an instructor in medicine in 1929 and progressed through the academic ranks to associate professor of medicine.[10] Among the rheumatologists who Bauer trained were Eric G.L. Bywaters,[7] Evan Calkins,[8] Alan S. Cohen,[12] John L. Decker,[13] Ephraim P. Engleman,[14] Irvin F. Hermann,[15] Joseph E. Levinson,[16] Hans Waine,[4] John R. Ward,[17] and Howard W. Weinberger.[18] Other prominent rheumatologists who trained as medical residents at the MGH under Bauer included K. Frank Austen,[19] J. Claude Bennett,[16] Edward D. Harris, Jr.,[16] Stephen M. Krane,[20] and Ralph C. Williams.[21] Austen appreciated that "Walter Bauer taught us to openly acknowledge what we did not know or understand so that we could learn and thereby benefit our patients."[10] Bauer believed that "scientific rigor and traditional humanitarianism are complementary aspects of medicine," and he advocated for integrating medical research with patient care and teaching in the academic medical center to advance medical knowledge.[22] Unfortunately, this is no longer the situation in many university hospitals now, where medical practitioners are excluded from the wards and clinics, and only full-time faculty are allowed to teach medical students, house staff, and fellows.

During World War II, Bauer served in the in the United States Army Medical Corps as Director of Medical Activities for the Eighth Service Command from August 1942 to August 1945, initially as a Lieutenant Colonel and later as a Colonel.[9,23] In this role, he established postgraduate medical education programs in US Army hospitals that "usually included weekly medical staff meetings, clinicopathologic conferences, clinical X-ray conferences, and biweekly hospital staff meetings. In addition, some of the medical services established journal clubs for reviewing the current medical literature."[23]

In February 1949, Bauer was 1 of 5 physicians with a special interest in rheumatic diseases who were invited by Philip Hench to visit the Mayo Clinic Rochester, Minnesota, to verify the "amazing" improvement of patients with rheumatoid arthritis following the administration of Compound E before this discovery was publicly reported.[24] Each of 2 rheumatoid arthritis patients received injections of Compound E on Monday afternoon and then were examined daily by the visiting physicians until that Friday. As Richard Freyberg later recalled, "During the course of 2 days, we watched them miraculously improve....One patient had been unable to sit down into a chair without assistance....He could sit and rise unassisted on the second day....By the third day, we saw improvement in the inflammation of the patients' joints....However, by the fourth and fifth days, these improvements disappeared, as did the patients' general feeling of well-being." Each of the 5 physicians presented their observations of the Mayo Clinic patients at the Seventh International Congress on Rheumatic Diseases, which took place in New York in 1949.[25] During his presentation, Bauer echoed the comment reportedly made by John Collins Warren in 1846, after the first public demonstration of ether anesthesia at MGH: "Gentlemen, this is no humbug."[24]

Shortly after his return from the Mayo Clinic and motivated by the dramatic responses of rheumatoid arthritis patients to Compound E that he had observed there, Bauer and his colleagues admitted a 21-year-old woman with persistently active juvenile-onset inflammatory arthritis despite treatment with aspirin and gold sodium thiomalate to the MGH in July 1949 for a therapeutic trial of adrenocorticotropic hormone (ACTH).[2] After 10 days of ACTH treatment, she reported that she "felt 'the best in one and one-half years.'" After she had received 3 weeks of ACTH treatment, "there was an unexpected increase in extension, passive but not active, of the proximal interphalangeal joints." However, within those 3 weeks, she developed characteristic clinical features of glucocorticoid toxicity. On the 130th day of treatment, she developed a "severe psychosis" that "necessitated immediate withdrawal of ACTH" and, within 2 weeks of stopping ACTH, she experienced a flare of joint inflammation that eventually subsided. Bauer and his colleagues concluded that "ACTH altered promptly and dramatically all the manifestations of disease activity, but the reversal was not complete (after 130 days), and the underlying disease process was not eradicated."

In 1951, Bauer was appointed chief of the medical services at the MGH and the Jackson professor of clinical medicine at Harvard Medical School.[9] Because, by that time, medical knowledge had expanded to the point that no individual could master all aspects, he created a medical service at the MGH comprised of 12 autonomous specialized units, each covering one of the medical specialties and consisting of full- and part-time physicians, clinical investigators, and basic scientists.[22,26] Each unit was to conduct basic laboratory research and to care for patients with diseases falling within that subspecialty. Interaction among all members of each unit was facilitated through weekly seminars in which clinical cases were presented and their pathophysiologic underpinnings discussed. In addition, physicians from each of the specialized units visited on the inpatient general medical wards and participated in teaching general internal medicine to medical students. To lead each unit, he appointed a physician who also had trained in a scientific discipline, such as biochemistry, biophysics, or physiology, and who displayed "superior competence in both fields."[26] Bauer had the foresight to select extremely talented recent graduates of the MGH medical residency program, such as Kurt J. Isselbacher, to head the gastrointestinal unit,[27] Morton N. Schwartz to head the infectious diseases unit,[28] and Lloyd H. Smith to head the endocrine unit.[29] Each of these physicians subsequently became a giant of American medicine. However, Bauer's leadership role on the medical services at MGH limited the time that he could devote to running the arthritis unit.

Bauer's clinical practice was limited to hospitalized patients, but patients came from all over to be cared for by Bauer.[9] Bauer's approach to treatment "was conservative in that he worked to conserve function and was skeptical of new and radical procedures," a characteristic that was continued by some of his disciples.[9] At that time, patients with rheumatoid arthritis were admitted to the MGH for a 6-month therapeutic program that included "absolute bed rest, high caloric diet, aspirin for analgesia, moist heat to affected joints, bed exercises intended to maintain and gain articular function and discussion concerning emotional factors." Because his "favorite drug" was aspirin, on a dinner and sightseeing cruise of San Francisco Bay during an annual meeting of the American Rheumatism Association, the walls of the ferryboat were covered with signs reading "Bauer's Aspirin" (instead of Bayer's Aspirin).[3] Stanley Cobb wrote that Bauer "steadfastly held out for the simple humanitarian values in practice. He really cared for his patients in both senses of the word. He looked after them meticulously and he supported them with his warm affection. He practiced and taught the art of quietly sitting down to take a comprehensive history so that he could learn what manner of man or woman his patient might be. He deemed it just as unscientific to neglect the emotional reactions as to omit the study of the chemistry of the body." Bauer believed that psychological factors were important in the pathogenesis of rheumatic diseases. In his 1947 presidential address to the American Rheumatism Association, he stated that "attention must be directed not only to the degree of structural impairment, but also to the personality as it relates to past capacities and flexibilities, as well as to its means of adapting to the specific disability. The emotional setting of the illness, the special meaning of the disability to the individual, and the past and present means used by the individual to manage or handle anxiety mobilized by disability, require particular attention."[30]

In addition to the American Rheumatism Association, of which he served as president between 1947 and 1948,[31] Bauer belonged to many medical organizations, including the American Association of Physicians, of which he served as president in 1959.[10,11] He was awarded honorary membership in several international organizations, including the Liga Argentina Contra el Reumatismo and the Sociedad Española de Reumatismo.[10] Bauer lectured and visited the countries of his former trainees.[32] He authored more than 170 scientific publications,[6] including the classic monographs on synovial fluid[33] and on rheumatoid arthritis.[34] In 1955, he was presented with the Heberden Medal in recognition of his research on rheumatic diseases.[7,10,11]

Bauer chain-smoked cigarettes[16] and died of complications of chronic lung disease on December 2, 1963, at age 65.[7,9] It was rumored that, because he was so beloved as a physician at the MGH, many of the colleagues who were treating him at the end of his life had difficulty allowing him to pass away. In his tribute to Bauer, John H. Knowles wrote that "he was one of the giants of our time and he left the MGH a better place in which to care for the sick. A salute to one who exemplified the highest qualities of the physician and added more to the MGH than he took away."[10] After Bauer's death, his former trainees honored him by establishing the Walter Bauer Lectureship in Rheumatology at the MGH and the Walter Bauer Scholarship Fund at Harvard Medical School.[10]

MARIAN WILKINS ROPES (1903–1994)

Marian Wilkins Ropes was born in Salem, Massachusetts, on December 1, 1903.[35,36] (**Fig. 2**) She received her bachelor of arts in chemistry from Smith College in 1924 and her master of science in chemistry from the Massachusetts Institute of Technology in 1926.[36] Following graduation, she worked as a technician in Aub's laboratory at the MGH.[37,38] This experience prompted her to pursue a career in medicine rather than one in chemistry. Because Harvard Medical School did not accept women, she applied only to the John Hopkins University School of Medicine and was accepted as 1 of 12 women in a class of 75 students.[35,39] After graduating from medical school in 1931, she completed an internship in medicine at Johns Hopkins Hospital.[35,39] James H. Means, then the chairman of the department of medicine at MGH, wanted to "get good women to apply" for postgraduate medical training at the MGH (a man well ahead of his time) and, in 1932, appointed Ropes as the first female resident in medicine at the MGH.[35] Upon completion of her residency in 1934, Bauer invited Ropes to join the Lovett Memorial Unit as a fellow, combining her research interest in chemistry with clinical work.

Ropes was the first female rheumatologist in the United States to have a productive academic career, both in research and clinical care. She spent over 40 years as a physician, teacher, and clinical investigator at the MGH and Harvard Medical School and was venerated by both colleagues and students "as a talented and intelligent clinician, researcher" and an educator.[35,36] She was an outstanding and clear-minded lecturer. In 1947, she was the first woman appointed as an assistant professor of clinical medicine at Harvard Medical School, and she became a consummate role model for women in medicine.[35,36] In 1940, she was the first woman elected to membership in the American Society of Clinical Investigation.[40] Ropes was promoted to associate clinical professor of medicine at Harvard Medical School in 1962. The following year, in 1963, she became the first woman elected president of the American Rheumatism

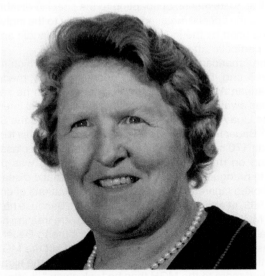

Fig. 2. Dr. Marian Wilkins Ropes.[35] (© 2023 President and Fellows of Harvard College. Marian Wilkins Ropes (Fielding). Memorial Minute, Harvard Medical School Office for Faculty Affairs.1994. https://fa.hms.harvard.edu/files/hmsofa/files/memorialminute_ropes_marian_w.pdf.)

Association.[41] Her alma mater, Smith College, presented her with an honorary doctor of science degree in 1965.[42] Both the American College of Physicians and the American Rheumatism Association (now the American College of Rheumatology) recognized her accomplishments by awarding Ropes the designation of master.[43,44] For many years, she was active in the national organization and in the Massachusetts chapter of the Arthritis Foundation, which established the Marian Ropes Award for Excellence in Arthritis Care and Leadership in her memory.[39]

Despite the availability of antirheumatic drugs such as antimalarials and gold salts, and the dramatic anti-inflammatory properties of glucocorticoids, Ropes was a strong proponent of conservative treatment for rheumatoid arthritis and advocated for the use of salicylates.[45] John A. Mills wrote that "Dr. Ropes was concerned about the impact of an illness on every aspect of a person's life. She believed strongly in the value of rest in the management of rheumatic disease but also strove to convince her patients that anything is possible if you try."[39] She favored a holistic approach to the management of patients with rheumatoid arthritis, emphasizing the importance of emotional support, rest, physical therapy, and a well-balanced diet with adequate intake of proteins, calcium, phosphorous, iron, and vitamins.[45]

Ropes became a professor emerita at Harvard Medical School in 1970 and remained as a member of the honorary staff at the MGH until her retirement in 1977.[35,36] However, despite retirement, she continued to interact with medical students, house staff, fellows, and her colleagues at the MGH.[35] Michelle A. Petri remembers when, as a medical student, she was introduced to Ropes at Rheumatology Grand Rounds. The rheumatology fellows whispered to her: "That is Marian Ropes!" Ropes was kind to her patients and to the medical students, house staff, and fellows she taught (M. Petri, 2023, personal communication). Ropes was Steven R. Goldring's first attending physician when he was a rheumatology fellow at the MGH. As he reminisces, "she was a kind, thoughtful and knowledgeable clinician with an immense experience in the diagnosis and management of rheumatic diseases. Although she had been involved in bench research, her real strengths were in her extensive clinical experience. She was an ideal attending for a fellow who was beginning his first year on the clinical service." (S.R. Goldring, personal communication). She was widely respected by everyone who came in contact with her. One can but imagine the impact that such a person had on the developing career of young trainees!

Ropes died on December 24, 1994, at age 91. There is no question that Ropes was a pioneer in American medicine who played an important role in breaking down barriers for women in medicine, not only at the MGH, at Harvard Medical School, and in the United States, but also around the world. As a physician, she was a role model for female trainees. She demonstrated that it was possible to be successful academically and still have a happy home life. She was so practical and down-to-earth, and Dwight R. Robinson recalled that Ropes' clothes always had to have pockets (M.A. Petri, personal communication). Ropes was known to have said: "The only thing that women need in medicine are pockets in women's clothes. Everybody laughs when I say that but it's the only thing I wish they would have done that they haven't. It's a crime."[35]

MAJOR SCIENTIFIC CONTRIBUTIONS

Given their close professional relationship, Bauer's and Ropes' scientific achievements can be considered together. Bauer's initial contributions to the field of rheumatology were studies on calcium and phosphorous metabolism in bone that were conducted in Aub's laboratory, in which Ropes worked as a technician.[46] In a series of 7 articles published between 1929 and 1932, he reported studies on calcium and phosphorous metabolism and excretion and their effects on trabecular bone in healthy individuals, those on a low calcium diet, pregnant women, patients with thyroid disease, and patients with hypoparathyroidism.[37,38,47–51] These studies were instrumental in elucidating the role of hormones in calcium and phosphorous metabolism and bone remodeling. He later extended these studies to include patients with rheumatoid arthritis, comparing them to patients with degenerative arthritis and healthy individuals as controls.[52] He showed that the rate of calcium metabolism and excretion was slightly increased in patients with rheumatoid arthritis. He postulated that even small effects over prolonged periods of time may contribute to the decalcification observed in patients with rheumatoid arthritis.[52]

Between 1930 and 1939, Bauer approached the study of rheumatism by conducting physiologic studies on synovial fluid and cartilage in cattle and dogs, and subsequently on human synovial fluid with Granville Allison Bennett at the Harvard Medical School.[53–57] He established a basic science group in association with Jerome Gross at the Massachusetts Institute of Technology, whom he subsequently recruited to the MGH to set up the Developmental Biology Laboratory, which generated fundamental advances in the understanding of connective tissue in health and disease.

In his seminal paper entitled "The *Diagnosis of the Various Arthritidies*" and published in the New England Journal of Medicine in 1939, Bauer highlighted the limitations of the then current rheumatological classifications of rheumatic diseases.[58] He suggested that a classification based on etiologic classification would be more useful to the practicing physician. Although not comprehensive, he classified joint diseases into: joint diseases of known etiology (infectious, neuropathic, metabolic, constitutional, and anaphylactic) joint diseases of unknown etiology (degenerative joint disease [primary or secondary], rheumatoid arthritis, and rheumatic fevers), and diseases of other skeletal structures of unknown etiology (tenosynovitis, bursitis, Dupuytren contracture, myositis, and fibrositis).[58] In this pivotal and influential paper, he stated that "rheumatoid spondylitis is classified as a form of rheumatoid arthritis because peripheral joints are often involved preceding or following the first symptoms referable to the spine." He believed strongly that "there is little justification for considering these patients as suffering from a different disease entity."[58] At the time, this was the prevailing thought regarding the clinical classification of spondyloarthritis. This concept was further supported in the 1957 book that he wrote with Charles L. Short and William A. Reynolds, in which they compared 252 rheumatoid arthritis patients with little or no spinal involvement with 41 cases of spondylitis.[34] Despite differences between the 2 groups such as earlier age of onset, more male involvement, and infrequent rheumatoid nodules in the spondylitic group, they concluded that "there is no justification in excluding those patients with spinal involvement, such an exclusion would render the series less than more representative of rheumatoid arthritis severe enough to warrant hospitalization."[58] It was not until the discovery of HLA-B27 that this controversy was finally resolved with the classification of spondyloarthritis as a distinct entity.[59,60] Some believe that such strong statements may have prevented the advancement of medicine and could possibly have tainted Bauer's legacy.[61] Regardless, in this landmark paper, Bauer meticulously described the signs and symptoms of the various rheumatic diseases and pointed out the limitations when using laboratory studies in their diagnosis. He highlighted the importance of careful clinical evaluation and observation in diagnosing rheumatic diseases, an important principle for all clinicians.[58]

Bauer collaborated closely with Ropes to study the physical and chemical properties of synovial fluid.[56,62] Because normal synovial fluid was present only in small amounts and was difficult to obtain by arthrocentesis, they effectively overcame this by using recently slaughtered young western cattle for their seminal studies of synovial fluid.[53] They demonstrated that, based on its chemical composition, synovial fluid was a dialysate of blood containing several other proteins such as mucin, albumin, and globin. They postulated that, in addition to its effects on colloid osmotic pressure and calcium concentration, mucin functioned as a lubricant and was important for maintaining joint function.[53,55–57,63] Further studies showed that mucin and polysaccharides in the synovial fluid were degraded by ascorbic acid and hydrogen peroxide.[64] Using dogs as an animal model, Bauer and Ropes were able to demonstrate the importance of molecular size and the lymphatic systems as essential factors involved in removing proteins from the joint and that exercise enhanced this process.[54] In this classic experiment, he was able to trace egg white or horse serum injected into the knees of dogs and monitor its appearance in blood and lymph obtained at regular intervals.

Other studies conducted by Ropes and Bauer included evaluation of the relationship between the erythrocyte sedimentation rate (ESR) and plasma proteins in patients with various inflammatory arthritidies, degenerative arthritis, and other non-rheumatological disorders.[65] They found a lack of correlation between ESR and plasma concentrations of fibrinogen and globulin, suggesting that variations in the plasma colloid with consequent changes in the charges of proteins of red cells contributed to variations in ESR. They also performed comparative electrophoretic analysis of synovial fluid proteins in inflammatory and traumatic effusions. The electrophoretic pattern of albumin and globulin correlated with the severity of disease and duration of the effusion.[66]

Ropes and Bauer published their comprehensive analysis of pathologic findings in synovial fluid from various joint diseases in 1953 in a book entitled *Synovial Fluid Changes in Joint Disease,* which became a classic (and even a bible) for rheumatologists of subsequent generations.[33] It is an extraordinary account of all the variations and perturbations that occur in synovial fluids from patients with various rheumatic diseases. This book set in motion the scientific study of synovial fluid as a mechanism by which to understand the pathophysiology of articular diseases, a process that has continued to this day in many laboratories around the world. It is unlikely, especially today, that a recent or current rheumatology fellow is aware of the Ropes test to detect the presence of synovial inflammation, whereby a clinician at the bedside could place a drop of synovial fluid into a tube of 1% acetic acid and observe the formation of a mucin clot appearing as a "tough, ropy mass," based upon the polymerization of hyaluronate.[33] In the presence of synovial fluid inflammation (regardless of the cause), the clot will dissipate rapidly causing the "surrounding solution" to become "very cloudy," and hence yield a positive Ropes test.

Bauer was a careful and meticulous observer who, with his colleague Charles L. Short, initiated long-term observational studies of the onset and course of rheumatoid arthritis. They established and followed a cohort of 293 rheumatoid arthritis patients at the MGH and compared and contrasted them to an equal number of carefully selected controls using statistical methods. They published their observations in 1957 in a book entitled: *Rheumatoid Arthritis: A Definition of the Disease and a Clinical Description Based on a Numerical Study of 293 Patients and Controls*, with William A. Reynolds as a co-author[34] In this book, they carefully recounted their experiences in treating and managing patients with rheumatoid arthritis from the 1930s to the 1950s and described all of the clinical manifestations that were known at that time.

In 1957, Ropes was instrumental, as committee chair, in developing the first diagnostic criteria for rheumatoid arthritis proposed by the American Rheumatism Association.[67] Given the difficult challenge of classifying rheumatoid arthritis at that time, the committee classified rheumatoid arthritis into three categories: (1) *definitive*; (2) *probable*; and (3) *possible* based upon the duration of signs and symptoms, and the presence of laboratory test abnormalities, radiographic findings, and characteristic histological features. Their classic publication, which subsequently was translated into French and Spanish, and became the benchmark for future classification and diagnostic criteria of other rheumatological disorders.[67] She later participated in developing the first set of preliminary criteria for clinical remission in rheumatoid arthritis, which were published in 1982.[68]

Later in her career, Ropes became interested in other rheumatologic diseases.[69,70] Her monograph on systemic lupus erythematosus is a classic, demonstrating her ability to use close observation to reach conclusions about cause and effect well before the implementation of biostatistical methodologies.[71] Petri credits one of her own earliest case-control studies to Ropes' observation that sulfa antibiotics led to flares of lupus disease activity. She recalls: "When I first came to Hopkins no one believed that Bactrim was a bad choice for people with lupus. I kept saying: Dr. Ropes said so! It led me to do the case-control study of antibiotics in lupus (and of course she was right!)." Petri recalls the impact of Ropes on her career: "I will never forget Dr. Ropes. It was reading her lupus monograph that convinced me to do lupus!" (M.A. Petri, personal communication).

Ropes was one of the few rheumatologists who supported limiting the use of glucocorticoids when treating patients with systemic lupus erythematosus, and she made important observations on the natural history of the disorder.[69] She advocated for the conservative management of lupus and often expounded on the dangers of glucocorticoid therapy, which were not widely accepted at that time.[69] She presented data suggesting that patients with systemic lupus erythematosus who were treated with glucocorticoids actually did worse than those who did not receive glucocorticoid therapy.[69] She was well aware of stress as a contributing risk factor to lupus flares. She was one of the first rheumatologists to emphasize that all patients with systemic lupus erythematosus were at increased risk for contracting infections and that infections contributed to their morbidity and mortality.[70,72]

SUMMARY

Walter Bauer was one of the most influential figures in the development of rheumatology as a medical subspecialty. He approached the study of rheumatic diseases both by careful clinical observation and description and by bringing basic scientists and clinicians together to study the "anatomy, chemical composition, and metabolism of connective tissue" in the laboratory.[8] Marian Wilkins Ropes was a pioneering woman in medicine; she was the first female medical resident at the MGH, the first woman appointed as an assistant professor of clinical medicine at Harvard Medical School, the first woman elected to membership in the American Society of Clinical Investigation, and the first woman elected president of the American Rheumatism Association. Both Bauer and Ropes were '*giants in rheumatology*' who made significant contributions to clinical medicine and scientific research and were great mentors and leaders of American rheumatology.

ACKNOWLEDGMENTS

The authors would like to thank those who provided anecdotes, perspectives, and insight into the lives and academic and research accomplishments of Walter Bauer and Marian Wilkins Ropes, including Dr George L. Cohen and Dr Steven R. Goldring, among others.

CONFLICTS OF INTEREST

The authors have nothing to disclose.

REFERENCES

1. Rudd E. Rheumatology and international health. International relations of the American Rheumatism Association. Arthritis Rheum 1972;15(4):417–24.
2. Giansiracusa JE, Ropes MW, Kulka JP, et al. The natural course of rheumatoid arthritis and the changes induced by ACTH. Am J Med 1951;10(4):419–38.
3. Engleman EP. The history of ACR: before 1970. In: Pisetsky DS, editor. The ACR at 75: a Diamond Jubilee. Hoboken (NJ): Wiley-Blackwell; 2009. p. 1–10.
4. Antonelli MJ, Calabrese CM, Calabrese LH, Kushner I. A brief history of American rheumatology. The Rheumatologist 2015.
5. Austen KF. Acceptance of the Kober medal: it only gets better. J Clin Invest 2004; 114(8):1177.
6. Walter Dr. Bauer of Harvard dead; physician, an authority on rheumatism, was 65. N Y Times 1963;1963:43.
7. Bywaters EGL. Walter Bauer, 1898-1963. Ann Rheum Dis 1964;23(2):170–1.
8. Calkins E. Walter Bauer, 1897-1963: in memoriam. Arthritis Rheum 1964;7:272–4.
9. Cobb S, Walter Bauer MD. 1898-1963. Psychosom Med 1964;26:103.
10. Massachusetts General Hospital. Bauer, Walter, MD. Catalog of arts & artifacts 2013; Available at: http://history.massgeneral.org/catalog/Detail.aspx?itemId=80 &searchFor=Picture/Portrait/Plaque. Accessed August 12, 2023.
11. Francis A. Countway Library of Medicine. Rare Books and Special Collection. Bauer, Walter, b. 1898. Papers, 1929-1960: A Finding Aid. Countway Library of Medicine, Center for the History of Medicine 2020; Available at: https://hollisarchives. lib.harvard.edu/repositories/14/resources/4557. Accessed August 12, 2023.
12. Alan Seymour Cohen, MD. 2018; Available at: https://www.bumc.bu.edu/camed/ 2018/05/09/alan-seymour-cohen-md/. Accessed August 12, 2023.
13. Office of NIH History and Stetten Museum. John L. Decker. NIH History 2023; Available at: https://onih.pastperfectonline.com/byperson?keyword=Decker% 2C%20John%20L. Accessed August 12, 2023.
14. Wofsy D. In memoriam: Ephraim P. Engleman, MD, 1911-2015. Arthritis Rheumatol 2015;67(11):2795–6.
15. Smukler NM. Division of rheumatology. In: Wagner Jr FB, editor. Thomas Jefferson university - Tradition and Heritage. Philadelphia, Pennsylvania: Thomas Jefferson University; 1989. p. 347–56.
16. Liang MH. History of the Robert Breck Brigham Hospital for Incurables. Boston: The Brigham and Women's Hospital, Inc.; 2013.
17. Devore C. A pioneer in rheumatology dies. The Daily Utah Chronicle 2004;2004.
18. Howard Weinberger, M.D. Los Angeles Times. February 4, 2007, 2007; Obituaries/Funeral Announcements, B13.
19. Drazen JM. Presentation of the 2004 Kober Medal to K. Frank Austen. J Clin Invest 2004;114(8):1174–6.
20. Dayer JM, Goldring MB, Goldring SR, et al. Tribute to Stephen M. Krane. J Bone Miner Res 2015;30(5):751–2.
21. Seo P. In Honor of Ralph C. Williams Jr., MD: rheumatologist & artist. The Rheumatologist 2021(July 2021).
22. Bauer W. The responsibility of the university hospital in the synthesis of medicine, science and learning. N Engl J Med 1961;265:1292–8.

23. Morgan HJ. Service commands. In: Havens Jr WP, editor. Activities of medical Consultants, vol. 1. Washington, DC: Office of the Surgeon General, Department of the Army; 1961. p. 71–141.
24. Freyberg R. Witness to a miracle: the initial cortisone trial: an interview with Richard Freyberg, MD. Interview by Mary Ellen Warner. Mayo Clin Proc 2001; 76(5):529–32.
25. The Seventh International Congress on Rheumatic Diseases. Ann Rheum Dis 1949;8(4):302–14.
26. Bauer W. Medicine in the teaching hospital of today and tomorrow. J Am Med Assoc 1959;171:1277–81.
27. Dienstag JL, Braunwald E, Podolsky DK, et al. Kurt J. Isselbacher. Memorial Minute 2019; Available at: https://fa.hms.harvard.edu/files/hmsofa/files/memorialminute_isselbacher_kurt_j.pdf. Accessed August 12, 2023.
28. Calderwood SB, Hooper DC, Karchmer AW, et al. Morton N. Swartz. Memorial Minute 2013; Available at: https://fa.hms.harvard.edu/files/memorialminute_swartz_morton_n.pdf. Accessed August 12, 2023.
29. Wachter RM, King TE Jr. A tribute to Lloyd Hollingsworth "Holly" Smith Jr. (1924–2018). J Clin Investig 2018;128(9):3649–50.
30. Bauer W. American Rheumatism Association presidential address: the challenge of adolescence. Ann Rheum Dis 1948;7(1):32–3.
31. American Rheumatism Association. Proceedings of the Annual Meeting, 1947. Ann Rheum Dis 1948;7(1):32–45.
32. Catoggio C, Catoggio LJ. Three(!) generations of rheumatologists: only in Argentina. J Can Rheumatol Assoc 2017;27(3):14–5.
33. Ropes MW, Bauer W. Synovial fluid changes in joint disease. Cambridge (MA): Harvard University Press; 1953.
34. Short CL, Bauer W, Reynolds WE. Rheumatoid arthritis: a definition of the disease and a clinical description based on a numerical study of 293 patients and controls, vol. 120. Cambridge (MA): Harvard University Press; 1957.
35. Krane S, Bennett JC, Ellis D, et al. Marian Wilkins Ropes (Fielding). Memorial Minute 1994; Available at: https://fa.hms.harvard.edu/files/hmsofa/files/memorialminute_ropes_marian_w.pdf. Accessed August 12, 2023.
36. National Library of Medicine. Dr. Marian Wilkins Ropes. Changing the face of medicine 2003; Available at: https://cfmedicine.nlm.nih.gov/physicians/biography_277.html. Accessed August 12, 2023.
37. Albright F, Bauer W, Ropes M, et al. Studies of calcium and phosphorus metabolism: IV. The effect of the parathyroid hormone. J Clin Invest 1929;7(1):139–81.
38. Aub JC, Bauer W, Heath C, et al. Studies of calcium and phosphorus metabolism: III. The effects of the thyroid hormone and thyroid disease. J Clin Invest 1929; 7(1):97–137.
39. Mills JA. Marian W. Ropes, MD, 1903–1994. Arthritis Rheum 1995;38(6):866.
40. Marr KA. The ownership paradox: nurturing continuity and change for the future ASCI. J Clin Invest 2019;129(12):5055–61.
41. American College of Rheumatology. ACR Past Presidents. 2022; Available at: https://assets.contentstack.io/v3/assets/bltee37abb6b278ab2c/blt92e5d62105dc8020/acr-past-presidents.pdf. Accessed August 12, 2023.
42. Smith College. Honorary degrees. 2023; Available at: https://www.smith.edu/about-smith/smith-history/honorary-degrees. Accessed August 12, 2023.
43. American College of Rheumatology. ACR Masters. 2023; Available at: https://assets.contentstack.io/v3/assets/bltee37abb6b278ab2c/bltd2fa473ae42d3566/acr-masters.pdf. Accessed August 12, 2023.

44. American College of Physicians. American College of Physicians Mastership Recipients 1923-present. 2023; Available at: https://www.acponline.org/sites/default/files/documents/about_acp/awards_masterships/masters.pdf. Accessed August 12, 2023.

45. Ropes MW. Conservative treatment in rheumatoid arthritis. Med Clin North Am 1961;45:1197–207.

46. Richardson EP, Aub JC, Bauer W. Parathyroidectomy in osteomalacia. Ann Surg 1929;90(4):730–41.

47. Albright F, Bauer W, Aub JC. Studies of calcium and phosphorus metabolism: VIII. The influence of the thyroid gland and the parathyroid hormone upon the total acid-base metabolism. J Clin Invest 1931;10(1):187–219.

48. Aub JC, Albright F, Bauer W, et al. Studies of calcium and phosphorus metabolism: VI. In hypoparathyroidism and chronic steatorrhea with tetany with special consideration of the therapeutic effect of thyroid. J Clin Invest 1932;11(1):211–34.

49. Bauer W, Albright F, Aub JC. Studies of calcium and phosphorus metabolism: II. The calcium excretion of normal individuals on a low calcium diet, also data on a case of pregnancy. J Clin Invest 1929;7(1):75–96b.

50. Bauer W, Aub JC. Studies of calcium and phosphorus metabolism. Xvi. The influence of the pituitary gland. J Clin Invest 1941;20(3):295–301.

51. Bauer W, Aub JC, Albright F. Studies of calcium and phosphorus metabolism : V. A study of the bone trabeculae as a readily available reserve supply of calcium. J Exp Med 1929;49(1):145–62.

52. Ropes MW, Rossmeisl EC, Bauer W. Calcium and phosphorus metabolism in rheumatoid arthritis and degenerative joint disease. J Clin Invest 1943;22(6):785–90.

53. Bauer W, Bennett GA, Marble A, et al. Observations on normal synovial fluid of cattle : I. The cellular constituents and nitrogen content. J Exp Med 1930;52(6):835–48.

54. Bauer W, Short CL, Bennett GA. The manner of removal of proteins from normal joints. J Exp Med 1933;57(3):419–33.

55. Rhinelander FW, Bennett GA, Bauer W. Exchange of substances in aqueous solution between joints and the vascular system. J Clin Invest 1939;18(1):1–13.

56. Ropes MW, Bennett GA, Bauer W. The origin and nature of normal synovial fluid. J Clin Invest 1939;18(3):351–72.

57. Warren CF, Bennett GA, Bauer W. The significance of the cellular variations occurring in normal synovial fluid. Am J Pathol 1935;11(6):953–68.

58. Bauer W. The diagnosis of the various arthritides. N Engl J Med 1939;221(14):524–33.

59. Brewerton DA, Hart FD, Nicholls A, et al. Ankylosing spondylitis and HL-A 27. Lancet 1973;1(7809):904–7.

60. Schlosstein L, Terasaki PI, Bluestone R, et al. High association of an HL-A antigen, W27, with ankylosing spondylitis. N Engl J Med 1973;288(14):704–6.

61. Ashrafi M, Ermann J, Weisman MH. Spondyloarthritis evolution: what is in your history? Curr Opin Rheumatol 2020;32(4):321–9.

62. Ropes MW, Rossmeisl EC, Bauer W. The origin and nature of normal human synovial fluid. J Clin Invest 1940;19(6):795–9.

63. Shaffer MF, Bennett GA. The passage of type Iii rabbit virulent pneumococci from the vascular system into joints and certain other body cavities. J Exp Med 1939;70(3):293–302.

64. Robertson WV, Ropes MW, Bauer W. The degradation of mucins and polysac-
    charides by ascorbic acid and hydrogen peroxide. Biochem J 1941;35(8–9):
    903–8.
65. Ropes MW, Rossmeisl E, Bauer W. The relationship between the erythrocyte sedi-
    mentation rate and the plasma proteins. J Clin Invest 1939;18(6):791–8.
66. Perlmann GE, Ropes MW, Kaufman D, et al. The electrophoretic patterns of pro-
    teins in synovial fluid and serum in rheumatoid arthritis. J Clin Invest 1954;33(3):
    319–25.
67. Ropes MW, Bennett GA, Cobb S, et al. Proposed diagnostic criteria for rheuma-
    toid arthritis. Ann Rheum Dis 1957;16(1):118–25.
68. Pinals RS, Baum J, Bland J, et al. Preliminary criteria for clinical remission in rheu-
    matoid arthritis. Bull Rheum Dis 1982;32(1):7–10.
69. Albert DA, Hadler NM, Ropes MW. Does corticosteroid therapy affect the survival
    of patients with systemic lupus erythematosus? Arthritis Rheum 1979;22(9):
    945–53.
70. Silverstein MD, Albert DA, Hadler NM, et al. Prognosis in SLE: comparison of Mar-
    kov model to life table analysis. J Clin Epidemiol 1988;41(7):623–33.
71. Ropes MW. Systemic lupus erythematosus. Cambridge (MA): Harvard University
    Press; 1976.
72. Ropes MW. Observations on the natural course of disseminated lupus erythema-
    tosus. Medicine (Baltim) 1964;43:387–91.

Eric Bywaters and Barbara Ansell

Founders of Modern Pediatric Rheumatology

Patricia Woo, CBE, FMedSci, MBBS, PhD, FRCP, FRCPCH[a],
Ross E. Petty, CM, MD, PhD, FRCPC[b],*

KEYWORDS

• Pediatric rheumatology • Founders • Canadian Red Cross Memorial Hospital
• Visionary development

THE CANADIAN RED CROSS MEMORIAL HOSPITAL, TAPLOW

The careers of Bywaters and Ansell, and the development of the field of pediatric rheumatology after the second world war are closely linked with the Canadian Red Cross Memorial Hospital built on the estate of Lord and Lady Astor in Cliveden, Taplow, Buckinghamshire, England (Appendix, **Tables 1** and **2**).[1] It was initially a hospital for the treatment of wounded Canadian servicemen in World War One. That hospital closed at the end of the war, but in 1939, supported by the Canadian Red Cross, the site was developed as a 600 bed hospital for treatment of Canadian sevicemen injured in the Second World War. In 1946 it was transferred to the National Health Service (NHS) to function as a general hospital with 100 beds allocated for the study and treatment of juvenile rheumatism. Of the 100 available beds, 4 were occupied by children with chronic arthritis, and the remainder by those with rheumatic fever at its opening in 1947.[2] Funding was available from the NHS, the Empire Rheumatism Council, the Medical Research Council and the Nuffield Trust. The Medical Research Council appointed Professor Bywaters as director of the unit while he still held the chair in Rheumatology at the Hammersmith Hospital in London. He recognized the need for a multidiscplinary team to address the challenges of dealing with childhood rheumatic diseases and recruited a stellar group of scientists and clinicians including pathologist Leonard Glynn and immunologist John Holborow. He recruited Barbara Ansell in 1952, his former registrar at the Hammersmith Hospital as consultant rheumatologist. This coincided with the emergence of interest in childhood rheumatic diseases in centers in Scandinavia, Europe, and the United States in particular. At the first major international meeting of pediatric rheumatologists in Park City, U.S.A., in 1977, Bywaters, who gave the opening address commented on the emergence of pediatric rheumatology as a specialty: "Pediatric rheumatology is one of the smallest, although I

a Rheumatology, University College Hospital, London, UK; b Division of Rheumatology, British Columbia's Children's Hospital, 4480 Oak Street, Vancouver British Columbia, Canada
* Corresponding author.
E-mail address: rosspetty2354@gmail.com

Rheum Dis Clin N Am 50 (2024) 93–101
https://doi.org/10.1016/j.rdc.2023.08.007
0889-857X/24/© 2023 Elsevier Inc. All rights reserved.

rheumatic.theclinics.com

Table 1	
Dr. Bywaters' honors	
Canada Gairdner International Award	1963
Heberden Orator	1966
Commander of the British Empire (CBE)	1975
Honorary Heberden Librarian, Royal College of Physicians	

would not say premature. I think I can say I saw it arrive, although I cannot specify its birthday or place, and I am damned if I can read the father's signature on the birth certificate."[2]

Over the course of many years, the program continued to flourish under Bywaters' direction. He recognized the serious nature of inflammatory eye disease in children with some types of chronic arthritis and recruited Mr Ken Smiley, ophthalmologist to study this problem and treat the affected children, in what may have been the earliest such collaboration. Mr George Arden and Mr Malcolm Swan, orthopedic surgeons joined the team to evaluate and treat children requiring surgical care including joint replacement surgery.

Taplow, as it was known by health professionals the world over, was a major focus of treatment and research in rheumatic diseases of childhood. The clinical spectrum of childhood rheumatic diseases was documented. Comparative clinical trials were carried out, often with international collaboration. The serious sequelae of prolonged illness including growth retardation, osteoporosis and amyloidosis were investigated and innovative therapies developed. The clinicians and scientists provided care for children from all over the United Kingdom, and many other countries. It was also the focus of postgraduate training of physicians from every continent. There are few pediatric rheumatologists working between the mid-sixties and the early nineties who did not receive at least part of their clinical experience at Taplow, and none who escaped its influence.

WHO WAS ERIC BYWATERS?

Eric George Lapthorne Bywaters was born in London in 1910. He graduated from the Middlesex Hospital Medical School in London in 1933 and was awarded a gold medal in pathology. He was appointed an Assistant Pathologist and studied cartilage and synovium with Sir Charles Dodds at the Courtauld Institute of Biochemistry in

Table 2	
Dr Ansell's honors	
M.D	1965
Heberden Orator	1971
Member, British Pediatric Association	1978
George Frederic Still Memorial Lecture	1981
Commander of the British Empire (CBE)	1982
James Spence Medal	1989
Honorary FRCS	1985

Fellow of three Medical Societies: Royal College of Surgeons; Royal College of Physicians; Royal College of Pediatrics and Child Health.

1934.[3] He worked with Dr Walter Bauer in Boston from 1937 to 1939 where, with his wife, Betty, he studied systemic lupus erythematosus. He returned to London in 1939, and took over the direction of the Rheumatism Unit at the Hammersmith Hospital and Postgraduate Medical School. He was both a pathologist and an able clinician and his career reflected the importance of communication between science and patient care. He studied "crush injury," renal failure caused by the release of myoglobin from crushed muscles incurred by soldiers and civilians during the war.[4] He collaborated with a Dutch physician, Willem J Kolff, who had developed a primitive dialysis machine and introduced renal dialysis as a management for myoglobin induced renal failure in the crush injury syndrome.[5]

At the inception of the NHS in 1947, Bywaters was appointed Director of the Special Unit of Juvenile Rheumatism at the Canadian Red Cross Memorial Hospital in Taplow. He was Clinical Head and Director of Research until his retirement in 1975 (**Fig. 1**).

Eric Bywaters was a keen observer of the clinical and pathologic evolution of his rheumatology patients while at the Hammersmith and pursued the same detailed documentation of clinical and pathologic followup of his patients continued at Taplow. His appreciation of the diagnostic challenges posed by patients whose clinical and pathologic presentation did not fulfill accepted diagnostic criteria with what he called "The Cheshire Cat syndrome," a phenomenon familiar to all rheumatologists, provide insight into his intellect and ability to "think outside the box." [6] The challenge of categorizing "Still Disease" was undertaken with Barbara Ansell and detailed in her MD thesis, and in his Heberden oration.[3] One of the central and ongoing discussions in pediatric rheumatology has been the matter of classification of chronic arthritis.

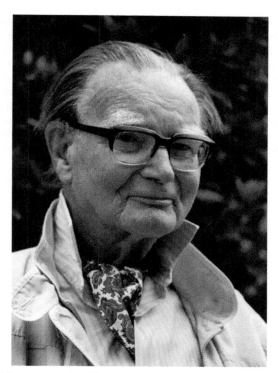

Fig. 1. Professor Eric Bywaters. (A. Dixon, Eric Bywaters 1910–2003, Rheumatology, Volume 42, Issue 8, August 2003, Pages 1025–1027, https://doi.org/10.1093/rheumatology/keg444.)

Bywaters and Ansell have addressed this question since the early 1960s. Their insights and arguments are informative. In his Heberden oration of 1966, Bywaters wrote: "Now there is some practical point in separating similar syndromes if prognosis or treatment differ or if pathogenesis is known to be different, but every patient has in one sense, his own disease, and treatment should always be individualized." This insight was presented decades before individualized medicine was even considered.

Bywaters traveled and lectured extensively. He grew a tree in his garden from seeds he collected on one of his travels from the tree under which Hippocrates is believed to have taught. He was an avid a gardener and a family man, holidaying with his wife and three daughters at their Welsh cottage (**Fig. 2**). He was an accomplished landscape and portrait painter in oils and watercolors. Aside from these hobbies he also had a major interest in medical history, was a collector of antique books, and was the Heberden librarian for the Royal College of Physicians for 20 years after his retirement in 1975. He was an enthusiastic skier and tennis player as well. He had a love of drawing from his days at medical school. A self-caricature is shown in **Fig. 3**.

Eric Bywaters died in 2003. He was pre-deceased in 1998 by Betty, his wife, who was a physiotherapist, and his collaborator.

WHO WAS BARBARA ANSELL?

Barbara Mary Ansell was born in Warwick, England, in 1923 (**Fig. 4**). She attended the University of Birmingham for medical training. She pursued training Pediatrics in Northampton, but then moved to London to work as a registrar in Medicine. She studied in Chicago for a year as an Eli Lily Fellow. On her return to England, she became a registrar in Medicine to Professor Bywaters at the Hammersmith Hospital. Her interest in becoming a cardiologist probably influenced her recruitment as a consultant rheumatologist to the MRC unit at Taplow by Bywaters. Rheumatic fever and its cardiac complications were still a major health problem and 1000 patients with rheumatic fever were admitted to Taplow between 1947 and 1955.[1] As the prevalence of rheumatic fever decreased, Ansell turned her attention to the plight of children with chronic arthritis who comprised an increasing portion of the children treated in the unit, and devoted her career to their investigation and care. She was impressed by the impact the disease had on the child's quality of life, and function, and the effect on the family. There was no effective treatment at the time, no center devoted to the care of children

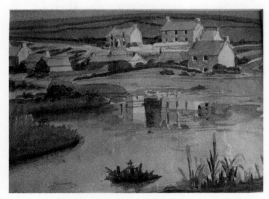

Fig. 2. Oil painting by Eric Bywaters. View from the family cottage in Wales. (Courtesy the Bywaters daughters.)

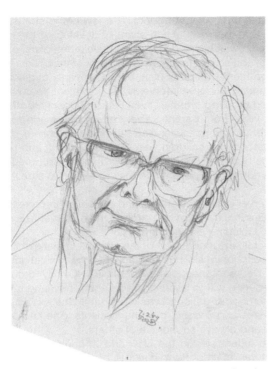

Fig. 3. Self-caricature by Eric Bywaters. (Courtesy the Bywaters daughters.)

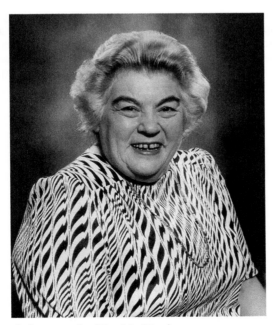

Fig. 4. Barbara Ansell. (Courtesy Prof Patricia Woo.)

with chronic arthritis in the United Kingdom, and few comprehensive programs any-where in the world. She took on the lion share of developing the clinical facility with a multidisciplinary team which included nurses, physiotherapists, occupational thera-pists, social workers, and school teachers. No aspect of the child's life was neglected. In today's terms, treatment was draconian, but the severity of disease and its myriad complications demanded intensive interventions. In-patient treatment of children with chronic arthritis often required months, even years of hospitalization. Distance often precluded frequent visits from parents. Every effort was made to provide the child with as normal a life as was possible. She did much to ensure that her colleagues and trainees, understood that children were not little adults, and required a different approach to management.[7] she understood the unique psychological, and develop-mental needs of the adolescent patient and their transition to care in the adult medical environment.[8]

A meticulous observer of family histories and clinical characteristics, Ansell and her colleagues were aware that genetics had a role in the pathogenesis of some childhood rheumatic diseases, including chronic arthritis.[9,10]

Her attention to detail, the recognition of the atypical, and insight into the role of ge-netics led to the description of siblings with a syndrome[11] which later became known as Chronic Infantile Neurocutaneous and Arthritis (CINCA) syndrome.[12]

She had a big presence with a booming voice and ready laughter. Her energy was phenomenal; her memory of patients was legendary. She expected much from her colleagues and trainees and, indeed, from her patients. She had a kind heart, was a generous colleague and always supportive of others.

Dr Ansell traveled extensively in the U.K. and throughout the world. She was a frequent guest lecturer at important national and international congresses. She became head of the Pediatric Rheumatology unit following its move from Taplow to Northwick Park in 1976.

Dr Ansell and her husband Dr Angus Weston (a general practitioner who pre-deceased her in 1991) were gracious and generous hosts to many visiting trainees and colleagues (**Fig. 5**). Barbara was an enthusiastic chef and dinner at their residence at Dumboyne in Stoke Poges was treasured by their guests. She was an opera enthu-siast, "Forza del Destino" being her favorite. Ansell had no children and often referred to her patients as "my special children." Barbara Ansell died in 2001.

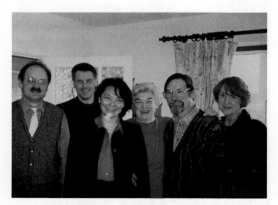

Fig. 5. Gathering of colleagues and trainees at the Ansell/Weston home. Left to right: Mark Walport, Taunton Southwood, Pat Woo, Barbara Ansell, Paul Bacon, Carol Black. (Courtesy Prof Patricia Woo.)

The Legacy

The careers of Eric Bywaters and Barbara Ansell were in many ways inseparable. Their contributions had a profound effect on the development of pediatric rheumatology. Their skills complemented each other: Bywaters the scientist and Ansell, the clinician collaborated effectively in patient care and in clinical and basic research.

Their establishment of a team of clinicians, allied health professionals, and basic scientists was remarkable in its day and has been a much emulated model since. Provision of training to hundreds of rheumatologist and pediatricians from all continents of the world, has done a great deal to establish the specialty of pediatric rheumatology world-wide. Recognition of the unique challenges presented by young patients did much to establish pediatric rheumatology as a specialty.

CLINICS CARE POINTS

- Define the need for different care for children and adolescents from that for adults.
- Interdiscipilinary team cares critical for optimal managment of rheumatic disease in chidlren and adolescents.

DISCLOSURE

The authors have no commercial or financial conflicts of interest. The authors have no funding sources related to this article.

ACKNOWLEDGMENTS

The authors are grateful to the daughters of Eric and Betty Bywaters for their cooperation and provision of **Figs. 2** and **3**.

REFERENCES

1. Ansell BM, Bywaters EGL, Spencer PE, et al. Looking back 1947-1985. Taplow, England: The Canadian Red Cross Memorial Hospital. Cliveden; 1997.
2. Bywaters EGL. The history of pediatric rheumatology. Arthritis Rheum 1977; 20(Suppl):145–52.
3. Bywaters EGL. Heberden Oration. Categorization in medicine: a survey of Still's disease. Ann Rheum Dis 1967;26:185–93.
4. Bywaters EG, Beall D. Crush injuries with impairment of renal function. Brit Med J 1941;1:427–32.
5. Bywaters EG, Joekes AM. The artificial kidney. Its clinical application in the treatment of traumatic anuria. Proc R Soc Med 1948;4:4520–5426.
6. Bywaters EG. The Cheshire Cat syndrome. Postgrad Med J 1968;44:20–2.
7. Ansell BM. How should pediatric rheumatology be delivered? Clin Exp Rheumatol 1994;12(Suppl):113–6.
8. Ansell BM, Chamberlain MA. Children with chronic arthritis: the management of transition to adulthood *Baillieres*. Clin Rheumatol 1998;12:363–73.
9. Ansell BM, Bywaters EG, Lawrence JS. A family study in Still's disease. Ann Rheum Dis 1962;3:243–52.
10. Clemens LE, Albert E, Ansell BM. Sibling pairs affected by chronic arthritis of childhood: evidence for a genetic predisposition. J Rheumatol 1988;12:108–13.

11. Ansell BM, Bywaters EG, Elderkin FM. Familial arthropathy with rash, uveitis and mental retardation. Proc Roy Soc Med 1975;68:584–5.
12. Prieur AM, Griscelli C, Lampert F, et al. A chronic infantile, neurocutaneous articular syndrome (CINCA) syndrome. A specific entity analyzed in 30 patients. Scand J Rheumatol 1987;66:57–68.

APPENDIX: SELECTED PUBLICATIONS

From among hundreds of publications including books (Rheumatic Diseases of Childhood by Barbara Ansell published in 1980), reviews, and editorials, the authors have selected several which document the breadth of expertise and often diverse interests of Bywaters and Ansell.

Bywaters EGL. The bursae of the body. Ann Rheum Dis 1965;24:215-218.

Bywaters EG. Still's disease in the adult. Ann Rheum Dis 1971;30:121-133.

Bywaters EG, Hamilton EB, Williams R. the spine in idiopathic haemochromatosis. Ann Rheum Dis 1971;30:453-465.

Bywaters EG. Historical aspects of ankylosing spondylitis. 1979;18:192-203.

Bywaters EG. The nosological status of "chronic secondary polyarthritis." Bull World Health Organ 1967;36:332-335.

Thompson M, Bywaters EG. Unilateral rheumatoid arthritis following hemiplegia. Ann Rheum Dis 1962;21:370-377.

Chambers RJ, Bywaters EG. Rubella synovitis. Ann Rheum Dis 1963;22:263-268.

Bywaters, EG. 50 years on: the crush syndrome. Brit Med J. 1990;301:1412-1415.

Thompson JM, Bluestone R, Bywaters EG, et al. Systemic muscle involvement in systemic sclerosis. Ann Rheum Dis 1969;28:281-288.

McMinn FJ, Bywaters EG. Differences between the fever of Still's disease and that of rheumatic fever. Ann Rheum Dis 1959;18:293-297.

Bywaters EGL. History of books and journals and periodicals in rheumatology. Ann Rheum Dis 1991;50:512-516.

Bywaters EG. George Frederic Still (1868-1941): his life and work. J Med Biogr 1994;2:1250131.

Ansell BM. Juvenile psoriatic arthritis. Balliere's Clin Rheumatol 1994;8:317-332

Shore A, Ansell BM. Juvenile psoriatic arthritis- analysis of 60 cases. J Pediatr 1982;100:529-535.

Ansell BM. Reactive arthritis/Reiter's syndrome in children. Clin Exp Rheumatol 1994;12:581-582.

Newman AJ, Ansell BM. Episodic arthritis in children with cystic fibrosis. J Pediatr 1974;94:594-596.

Palmer RG, Kanski JJ, Ansell BM. Chlorambucil in the treatment of intractable uveitis associated with juvenile chronic arthritis. J Rheumatol 1985;12:967-970.

Schnitzer TJ, Ansell BM. Amyloidosis in juvenile chronic polyarthritis. Arthritis Rheum 1970;20 (suppl) 245-252.

Ansell BM, Nasseh GA, Bywaters EG. Scleroderma in childhood. Ann Rheum Dis 1976;35:189-197.

Ansell BM. Acute arthritis in children. Curr Med Res Opin. 19745;9:594-595.

Ansell BM. Uncommon radiological features of chronic arthritis in childhood. A review. J Roy Soc Med 1981;74:904-908.

Ansell BM, Hanna DB, Stoppard M. Naproxen absorption in children. Curr Med Res Opin. 1995;3:46-50.

Allen RC, St.Cyr C, Maddison PJ, et al. Overlap connective tissue syndromes. Arch Dis Child 1986;61:284-288.

Lewkonia RM, Ansell BM. Articular hypermobility simulating chronic rheumatic disease. Arch Dis Child. 1988;58:988-992.

Ansell BM, Bywaters EG. Growth in Still's disease. Ann Rheum Dis. 1956;15:295-309.

Byron MA, Jackson J, Ansell BM. Effect of different corticosteroid regimens on hypothalamic-pituitary axis and growth in juvenile chronic arthritis. J Roy Soc Med 1983;76:452-457.

Earley A, Cuttica RJ, McCullough C, et al. Triamcinolone into the knee joint in juvenile chronic arthritis. Clin Exp Rheumatol 1988;6:153-155.

Loftus JK, Reeve J, Hesp R, et al. Deflazacort in juvenile chronic arthritis. J Rheumatol Suppl 1993;37:40-42.

Wynne-Davies R, Hall C, Ansell BM. Spondylo-epiphyseal dysplasia tarda with progressive arthropathy. A "New" disorder of autosomal recessive inheritance. J Bone Joint surg (Br) 1982;64:442-4456.

Davies UM, Rooney M, Preese MR, et al. Treatment of growth retardation in juvenile chronic arthritis with recombinant human growth hormone. J Rheumatol 1994;21:153-158.

Ansell BM, Arden GF, McLennan I. Valgus knee deformities in children with juvenile chronic polyarthritis treated by epiphyseal stapling. Arch Dis Child 1970;45:388-392.

Witt JD, Swann M, Ansell BM. Total hip replacement for juvenile chronic arthritis. J Bone Joint Surg. 1992;73:770-773.

Schaller JG, Johnson GD, Holborow EJ, et al. The association of antinuclear antibodies with chronic iridocyclitis in juvenile rheumatoid arthritis (Still's disease). Arthritis Rheum 1974;17:409-4126.

Fink CW, Ansell BM, Wood PHN. Juvenile arthritis in England. A long-term followup. Arthritis Rheum 1980;23: 673.

H. Ralph Schumacher

Joshua F. Baker, MD, MSCE[a,b,c],*, Daniel G. Baker, MD[d]

KEYWORDS

- Biopsy • Inflammatory response • Osteoarthritis • Rheumatology
- Rheumatoid arthritis

KEY POINTS

- Dr. Schumacher utilized synovial biopsy, electron microscopy, and other tools to describe many of the most common forms of arthritis.
- He was dedicated to education and mentorship both at his own institution but also globally, mentoring scholars from around the world.
- Through research and education, his work has shaped current practice in many ways, particularly with regard to common conditions like gout.

BACKGROUND AND INTRODUCTION

The definition of a giant in this context is "a person of exceptional importance and reputation". H. Ralph Schumacher certainly fits this definition in the field of rheumatology. His research, global mentorship, and dedication to patient care transformed the field of rheumatology and continues to benefit patients worldwide.

Dr Schumacher was born in Montreal and became a Philadelphia area native. He was star basketball player at Ursinus college where he chose medicine as a profession with his usual dedication and commitment. He earned his medical degree at the University of Pennsylvania. During this time, he spent a summer working at a Native American hospital in Oklahoma and a Summer doing research on nutrition in Guatemala—experiences that stuck with him throughout his career.

He did his residency in Los Angeles at the Wadsworth Veteran's Affairs Medical Center and the University of California Los Angeles. He chose rheumatology because it was so new and he believed he could make a difference (it seems he was right). He did a fellowship in rheumatology at Robert B. Brigham hospital and a fellowship in pathology at the Peter B. Brigham hospital where he learned to use the electron microscope. He interrupted his early training to serve in the Air Force in California as a Staff

[a] Corporal Michael J. Crescenz VA Medical Center, Philadelphia, PA, USA; [b] Perelman School of Medicine, University of Pennsylvania, Philadelphia, PA, USA; [c] Department of Biostatistics, Epidemiology, and Informatics, Perelman School of Medicine, University of Pennsylvania, Philadelphia, PA, USA; [d] Kira Biotech Pty Ltd, Fortitude Valley, Queensland, Australia
* Corresponding author. 5th Floor White Building, 3400 Spruce Street, Philadelphia, PA 19104.
E-mail address: Joshua.Baker@pennmedicine.upenn.edu

Rheum Dis Clin N Am 50 (2024) 103–111
https://doi.org/10.1016/j.rdc.2023.08.008
0889-857X/24/Published by Elsevier Inc.

rheumatic.theclinics.com

Physician during which time he was the only rheumatologist. After his training, he practiced for the rest of his career at the Philadelphia VA Medical Center and as a faculty member at the University of Pennsylvania for more than 50 years. Although he spent most of his long career at a single institution, the effect of his career has been felt globally.

Dr Schumacher is best known for what has been called his "bench to bedside and back" approach to research. He was a leader in the use of light microscopy and electron microscopy—tools he used to describe the cellular underpinnings of clinical presentations he observed in the clinic. Perhaps what he is most known for is his characterization of crystal diseases and their associated inflammatory responses. In addition, he embraced clinical research and the rigorous study of new approaches to management.

Dr Schumacher highly valued cooperation and collaboration. His guiding philosophy may be best described in his own words—words that he used to describe images from electron micrographs: "reach out, stick together, cooperate, depart from the routine, hug, take action, be flexible, try to heal, be a bit mysterious and not afraid to be puzzled, be productive, and band together to achieve." Those who worked with him noted that he never shied away from an interesting research question and loved to speculate about new questions, studies, and hypotheses. He was also an enthusiastic and gifted teacher and speaker and shared his observations and knowledge widely and with great effect. His dedication and commitment to advancing knowledge kept him working until his death from amyotrophic lateral sclerosis at the age of 83 years.

Although he was certainly a highly productive physician-scientist, it is worth noting that Dr Schumacher was also an active person in his personal life. He never lost his love for basketball and played well into his 50s. He was also an avid gardener. He and his wife Elizabeth created a stunning award-winning garden in their terraced backyard, which served as a lovely and frequent venue for collegial gatherings and which was eventually listed in the Archives of American Gardens at the Smithsonian. He and Elizabeth also wrote a book on gardening entitled "*The Idiosyncratic Garden, How to create and enjoy a personalized garden*." Dr Schumacher also loved to travel, which he did frequently and widely. His family remembers his sense of humor, his love of puns, poems, and word play, as well as his love of art, stamps, sports, and languages.

One might say that Dr Schumacher's job was his favorite hobby. The following is a summary of not only the scientific contributions of H. Ralph Schumacher but also his leadership in advancing the field of Rheumatology both at home and abroad.

Major Scientific Contributions

Dr Schumacher's scientific accomplishments span 6 decades and include impactful work within basic science and clinical research. Although it is impossible to summarize in any detail the hundreds of publications that carried his name, we aimed to briefly discuss some key areas that help to illustrate his interests and impact.

Dr Schumacher is known for his "bench to bedside and back" approach to research. He was a leader in the use of light microscopy and electron microscopy, and he used those tools in both synovial fluid and synovium to describe the cellular underpinnings of presentations he observed in the clinic. He performed countless synovial biopsies and synovial fluid analyses, allowing for deep characterization of synovial pathology in several conditions ranging from crystal diseases to osteoarthritis (OA) to inflammatory arthritis. Perhaps what he is most known for is his characterization of crystal diseases and their associated inflammatory responses. Importantly, he brought that knowledge back to the clinic embracing clinical research and the rigorous study of new approaches to management.

TOOLS OF HIS TRADE

Dr Schumacher's passion was to describe the presentation and synovial characteristics of patients with rheumatic diseases using synovial analysis paired with synovial biopsies. Early in his career, Dr Schumacher was a pioneer and early expert in the use of synovial biopsy to evaluate different types of arthritis and described the method of performing synovial biopsies in the New England Journal of Medicine.[1] In the 60s he was the first, to our knowledge, to describe the synovitis associated with pseudogout and hemochromatosis[2,3] as well as a long list of other conditions.[4,5] Of great import was also the characterization of the features of normal synovium.[6] In these studies, he described the clinical presentations in great detail and correlated with the description of tissue from synovial biopsy specimens using light and electron microscopy. This unique combination of tools allowed a detailed description of not only gross pathology but also details of cell-cell interactions, synovial lining cell types and function, and clues to physiologic function (eg, lack of a basement membrane in synovial lining).

Over his career, Dr Schumacher first described the articular manifestations of common rheumatic diseases including systemic lupus, scleroderma, and polymyalgia rheumatica, finding that these forms of arthritis were generally less inflammatory than rheumatoid arthritis but were observed to have more significant vascular involvement.[7–10]

Dr Schumacher was widely regarded as the leading expert in synovial fluid analysis, particularly with regard to evaluating crystal diseases (**Figs. 1** and **2**). He described the

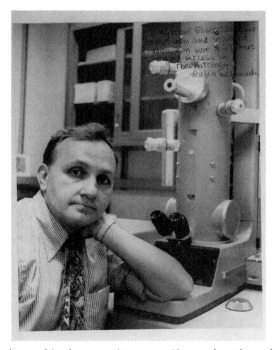

Fig. 1. Dr Schumacher at his electron microscope. Picture thought to be taken by Eliseo Pascual when he was a fellow in his laboratory. (Dr. H. Ralph Schumacher, Jr. at his electron microscope. Picture used with permission from Elizabeth Schumacher.)

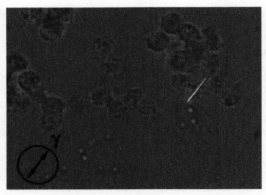

Fig. 2. A picture of a monosodium urate crystal taken by Dr Schumacher.

appearance of many different types of crystals, including monosodium urate, calcium pyrophosphate dihydrate (CPPD), calcium oxalate, and calcium hydroxyapatite (HA) crystals and also described the appearance of other substances that could be found in synovial fluid samples such as cholesterol crystals, lipid droplets, talc particles, and corticosteroid crystals.[11] He recognized and preached the importance of synovial analysis in diagnosis and treatment. He also demonstrated the poor reproducibility of this process across laboratories early on, an observation that fueled his desire to provide education and better standardize the utilization of this tool in clinical practice among rheumatologists.[12]

CRYSTAL-INDUCED ARTHROPATHIES

Dr Schumacher is perhaps most well-known for his work in crystal-induced arthropathies, most notably gout. His work in this disease spans decades and covers basic pathophysiology to clinical trials. Early in his career he evaluated the neutrophil changes occurring in response to monosodium urate crystals including the intravascular degranulation of neutrophils[13–15] and described the exacerbating effect of exercise on urate-related inflammation in a dog model of gout.[15,16] His early observations served as an important foundation for the understanding of the pathophysiology of the disease, the clinical presentation, and the response to commonly used therapies such as colchicine.

His work also described the pathology associated with other crystal diseases such as hydroxyapatite disease[17] and pseudogout, as well as the role of crystals in OA.[18–21] His work with Dan McCarty and Joe Hollander described the appearance of CPPD crystals in synovial fluid and ultimately expanded our understanding of the pathology of pseudogout. In addition, with observations made over multiple decades, he demonstrated a close association between calcium crystals (HA and CPPD) and the severity of osteoarthritis, which has led to a better understanding of their role in the progression of the joint degeneration in OA.

His use of electron microscopy was unique in the field and gave unique perspective on crystal formation, size, structure, and protein-crystal interactions to help explain different presentations of crystal-induced arthritis.

In addition to extensive work describing the histologic manifestations of crystal arthritis, Dr Schumacher was intent on making his research clinically relevant. He thus played an early role in defining the course of clinical research in this disease.

He described the seasonality associated with gout,[22] explored associations between gout and cardiovascular diseases,[23,24] helped to develop clinical and patient-reported outcomes for the disease,[25–27] and participated in several clinical trials evaluating both treatments for acute gout as well as urate-lowering therapies.[28–31] For example, he led a trial of rilonacept for the prevention of gout during urate lowering therapy[32] (it worked) and high-dose Celebrex for the management of acute gout (it also worked).[33]

CLINICAL RESEARCH AND CLINICAL PRACTICE

Throughout his career, but perhaps most notably toward his later years, Dr Schumacher played a role in shaping the management of other common forms of arthritis through his involvement in several clinical research studies and clinical trials. For example, he was involved in a study evaluating the performance of the 1987 American College of Rheumatology classification criteria for rheumatoid arthritis.[34] He also participated in clinical trials evaluating the effectiveness of etanercept in reactive and undifferentiated arthritis (there was some benefit)[35] and the value of tart cherry juice in osteoarthritis (there was no benefit).[36] Finally, he was involved in educational initiatives and wrote many high-impact clinical reviews on several rheumatologic and systemic diseases and conditions with the aim of promoting better clinical care.[37–40] He also frequently published editorials in order to stimulate meaningful discussion around current practice.[41]

Global Mentoring and Education

Over his career, Dr Schumacher mentored more than 200 scholars from more than 30 countries across the globe. Visiting scholars were common in his laboratory and came from places such as Venezuela, Ecuador, Brazil, Argentina, Chile, Mexico, Columbia, Thailand, China, Taiwan, and Japan, among others. He believed it was important to widely disseminate rheumatologic research and best clinical practices around the globe, and he was deliberate in his efforts, not only by providing his laboratory and resources to train young rheumatologists but also by visiting and spending time with his foreign trainees helping them establish rheumatology centers of excellence in their own home countries. Central America and South America were frequently visited countries, and he established a Pan American League of Associations for Rheumatology (PANLAR)-Schumacher Award to support junior investigators in Latin America. He also taught countless fellows, students, residents, and junior faculty at the University of Pennsylvania both in clinical care and in research. His name lives on at the University of Pennsylvania through research awards for fellows and junior faculty.

We asked people who worked with Dr Schumacher over his career to share some of the most important features of his personality as a mentor and educator. He was an introvert who was not into "chit-chat" but was a vigorous advocate for his mentees and found great reward from observing their intellectual development and career growth. Perhaps his most notable personality trait for mentees was his innate and insatiable curiosity. He was able to find interesting questions in even the most mundane or routine clinical scenarios. He found many things interesting, was highly supportive of new ideas, and constantly asked the question "why?" Dr Schumacher was also known to say "I don't know" unashamedly. He used these moments to encourage thoughtful consideration of the ongoing knowledge gaps in the field and to propose new studies, often encouraging those around him to take on the work of addressing unanswered questions.

National and International Leadership

Dr Schumacher was a leader in the field in multiple areas across the United States and across the globe. He served several roles within the American College of Rheumatology (ACR) including acting as the Chairman of the Educational Committee. He also ran highly attended workshops on crystal analysis at the ACR for many years. He helped to craft questions for the rheumatology boards and served on the editorial board for more than 20 journals. He helped to organize networks of rheumatologists within the Veterans Affairs including helping to found the VA Rheumatology Consortium (VARC). Finally, he was an active member of "Outcome Measures in Rheumatology" (OMERACT) in developing outcome measures for gout.

A critical contribution was his founding of the Journal of Clinical Rheumatology, with the goal of publishing clinically oriented work from around the globe. He served as Editor-in-Chief for 23 years. This journal aims to help clinicians by providing practical information directly relevant to clinical care in an easily accessible format.

In recognition of his leadership, Dr Schumacher was given several prestigious awards during his career, including the Hench Award of the Association of Military Surgeons and the ACR Klemperer Lectureship Award.

Impact on Current Practice

Some of the common acts that we take for granted in clinical practice stem from Dr Schumacher's work. Now a foundational skill, the art of crystal analysis, was characterized and emphasized by Dr Schumacher over the course of his career. He described the appearance of crystals and other substances that could be found in synovial fluid and disseminated these descriptions widely.[11] These observations are still used today in textbooks and countless teaching materials to help train young physicians in this important skill. With his frequent travel, he helped to establish numerous synovial fluid laboratories across the world.

Perhaps most well-known for his work in gout, Dr Schumacher was involved in many key clinical studies evaluating the management of gout. As noted, he helped to develop appropriate outcomes for gout, participated in large clinical trials, and wrote numerous reviews discussing the diagnosis and management of gout.[42,43]

Dr Schumacher performed countless synovial biopsies and described synovial tissue in many diseases including gout, rheumatoid arthritis, reactive arthritis, scleroderma, and polymyalgia rheumatica, among others. He provided detailed histologic and clinical descriptions of important conditions in rheumatology, including things such as scurvy, eosinophilic fasciitis, ochronosis, hepatitis-related arthritis, hypertrophic pulmonary osteoarthropathy, pigmented villonodular synovitis, Lyme disease, pancreatic osteoarthropathy, and sickle cell disease, among others. The foundational studies provided key insights at a time when the field was starting to understand new conditions and consider new treatments and management strategies.

Beyond his research efforts, Dr Schumacher was a key figure in the early education of the next generation of rheumatologists. His educational process and enthusiasm for the effective dissemination of information helped to move practice patterns across the globe. Similarly, he mentored countless physician-scientists (including these investigators) and helped launch careers that had far-reaching, if intangible, effects on the practice of rheumatology.

Dr Schumacher may not only have influenced *how* we practice rheumatology but also *where*. His engagement and influence on the global stage helped shape and improve rheumatology care across the world through superb educational talks, close communication with many international collaborators, engagement in international communities, and his love of travel, particularly in a time when "virtual" talks and conferences did not exist.

SUMMARY

In summary, Dr Schumacher was a force in rheumatology for more than half a century through his multiple roles as a researcher, clinician, mentor, and educator. He is not likely to be soon forgotten by the rheumatology community; however, it is hoped that this chapter can provide a faithful recollection that will help bring his memory to life for some and that rings true to those who knew him and learned from him.

CONFLICTS OF INTEREST

The authors have nothing to disclose.

FUNDING

Dr Baker is supported by a VA Clinical Science Research & Development Merit Award (CX001703) and a Rehabilitation Research & Development Merit Award (RX003644).

ACKNOWLEDGMENTS

We would like to thank those who provided anecdotes, perspectives, and insights into Dr Schumacher's life and career, including Joan Von Feldt, Gilda Claybourne, Janet Dinnella, and Ted Lally, among others. In particular, we would like to thank Elizabeth Schumacher, who provided her thoughtful perspectives as well as the picture featured in the chapter.

REFERENCES

1. Schumacher HR Jr, Kulka JP. Needle biopsy of the synovial membrane–experience with the Parker-Pearson technic. N Engl J Med 1972;286(8):416–9.
2. Schumacher HR Jr. The synovitis of pseudogout: electron microscopic observations. Arthritis Rheum 1968;11(3):426–35.
3. Schumacher HR Jr. Hemochromatosis and Arthritis. Arthritis Rheum 1964;7: 41–50.
4. Bevelaqua FA, Hasselbacher P, Schumacher HR. Scurvy and hemarthrosis. JAMA 1976;235(17):1874–6.
5. Schumacher HR Jr. Articular manifestations of hypertrophic pulmonary osteoarthropathy in bronchogenic carcinoma. Arthritis Rheum 1976;19(3):629–36.
6. Singh JA, Arayssi T, Duray P, et al. Immunohistochemistry of normal human knee synovium: a quantitative study. Ann Rheum Dis 2004;63(7):785–90.
7. Chou CT, Schumacher HR Jr. Clinical and pathologic studies of synovitis in polymyalgia rheumatica. Arthritis Rheum 1984;27(10):1107–17.
8. Chou CT, Schumacher HR. Polymyalgia rheumatica. Compr Ther 1983;9(9):33–7.
9. Schumacher HR Jr. Joint involvement in progressive systemic sclerosis (scleroderma): a light and electron microscopic study of synovial membrane and fluid. Am J Clin Pathol 1973;60(5):593–600.
10. Labowitz R, Schumacher HR Jr. Articular manifestations of systemic lupus erythematosus. Ann Intern Med 1971;74(6):911–21.
11. Kahn CB, Hollander JL, Schumacher HR. Corticosteroid crystals in synovial fluid. JAMA 1970;211(5):807–9.

12. Schumacher HR Jr, Sieck MS, Rothfuss S, et al. Reproducibility of synovial fluid analyses. A study among four laboratories. Arthritis Rheum 1986;29(6):770–4.

13. Schumacher HR, Phelps P. Sequential changes in human polymorphonuclear leukocytes after urate crystal phagocytosis. An electron microscopic study. Arthritis Rheum 1971;14(4):513–26.

14. Schumacher HR, Agudelo CA. Intravascular degranulation of neutrophils: an important factor in inflammation? Science 1972;175(4026):1139–40.

15. Schumacher HR, Phelps P, Agudelo CA. Urate crystal induced inflammation in dog joints: sequence of synovial changes. J Rheumatol 1974;1(1):102–13.

16. Agudelo CA, Schumacher HR, Phelps P. Effect of exercise on urate crystal-induced inflammation in canine joints. Arthritis Rheum 1972;15(6):609–16.

17. Bonavita JA, Dalinka MK, Schumacher HR Jr. Hydroxyapatite deposition disease. Radiology 1980;134(3):621–5.

18. Schumacher HR Jr. Crystals, inflammation, and osteoarthritis. Am J Med 1987; 83(5A):11–6.

19. Schumacher R Jr. The role of inflammation and crystals in the pain of osteoarthritis. Semin Arthritis Rheum 1989;18(4 Suppl 2):81–5.

20. Schumacher HR Jr. Synovial inflammation, crystals, and osteoarthritis. J Rheumatol Suppl 1995;43:101–3.

21. Nalbant S, Martinez JA, Kitumnuaypong T, et al. Synovial fluid features and their relations to osteoarthritis severity: new findings from sequential studies. Osteoarthritis Cartilage 2003;11(1):50–4.

22. Schlesinger N, Gowin KM, Baker DG, et al. Acute gouty arthritis is seasonal. J Rheumatol 1998;25(2):342–4.

23. Baker JF, Krishnan E, Chen L, et al. Serum uric acid and cardiovascular disease: recent developments, and where do they leave us? Am J Med 2005;118(8): 816–26.

24. Krishnan E, Baker JF, Furst DE, et al. Gout and the risk of acute myocardial infarction. Arthritis Rheum 2006;54(8):2688–96.

25. Taylor WJ, Singh JA, Saag KG, et al. Bringing it all together: a novel approach to the development of response criteria for chronic gout clinical trials. J Rheumatol 2011;38(7):1467–70.

26. Singh JA, Taylor WJ, Simon LS, et al. Patient-reported outcomes in chronic gout: a report from OMERACT 10. J Rheumatol 2011;38(7):1452–7.

27. Schumacher HR, Taylor W, Edwards L, et al. Outcome domains for studies of acute and chronic gout. J Rheumatol 2009;36(10):2342–5.

28. Schumacher HR Jr, Becker MA, Wortmann RL, et al. Effects of febuxostat versus allopurinol and placebo in reducing serum urate in subjects with hyperuricemia and gout: a 28-week, phase III, randomized, double-blind, parallel-group trial. Arthritis Rheum 2008;59(11):1540–8.

29. Terkeltaub RA, Schumacher HR, Carter JD, et al. Rilonacept in the treatment of acute gouty arthritis: a randomized, controlled clinical trial using indomethacin as the active comparator. Arthritis Res Ther 2013;15(1):R25.

30. Schumacher HR Jr, Boice JA, Daikh DI, et al. Randomised double blind trial of etoricoxib and indometacin in treatment of acute gouty arthritis. BMJ 2002; 324(7352):1488–92.

31. Schlesinger N, Detry MA, Holland BK, et al. Local ice therapy during bouts of acute gouty arthritis. J Rheumatol 2002;29(2):331–4.

32. Schumacher HR Jr, Sundy JS, Terkeltaub R, et al. Rilonacept (interleukin-1 trap) in the prevention of acute gout flares during initiation of urate-lowering therapy:

results of a phase II randomized, double-blind, placebo-controlled trial. Arthritis Rheum 2012;64(3):876–84.

33. Schumacher HR, Berger MF, Li-Yu J, et al. Efficacy and tolerability of celecoxib in the treatment of acute gouty arthritis: a randomized controlled trial. J Rheumatol 2012;39(9):1859–66.

34. Levin RW, Park J, Ostrov B, et al. Clinical assessment of the 1987 American College of Rheumatology criteria for rheumatoid arthritis. Scand J Rheumatol 1996; 25(5):277–81.

35. Flagg SD, Meador R, Hsia E, et al. Decreased pain and synovial inflammation after etanercept therapy in patients with reactive and undifferentiated arthritis: an open-label trial. Arthritis Rheum 2005;53(4):613–7.

36. Schumacher HR, Pullman-Mooar S, Gupta SR, et al. Randomized double-blind crossover study of the efficacy of a tart cherry juice blend in treatment of osteoarthritis (OA) of the knee. Osteoarthritis Cartilage 2013;21(8):1035–41.

37. Baker DG, Schumacher HR Jr. Acute monoarthritis. N Engl J Med 1993;329(14): 1013–20.

38. Schumacher HR, Pessler F, Chen LX. Diagnosing early rheumatoid arthritis (RA). What are the problems and opportunities? Clin Exp Rheumatol 2003;21(5 Suppl 31):S15–9.

39. Schumacher HR, Chen LX, Glick L. Evaluation of a knee and shoulder arthrocentesis training program for primary care providers. J Rheumatol 2008;35(10): 2083–4.

40. Schumacher HR, Chen LX, Mandell BF. The time has come to incorporate more teaching and formalized assessment of skills in synovial fluid analysis into rheumatology training programs. Arthritis Care Res 2012;64(9):1271–3.

41. Schumacher HR. Are we being open enough to all approaches to therapy of rheumatoid arthritis? J Clin Rheumatol 2013;19(4):167–71.

42. Schlesinger N, Schumacher HR Jr. Update on gout. Arthritis Rheum 2002;47(5): 563–5.

43. Baker JF, Schumacher HR. Update on gout and hyperuricemia. Int J Clin Pract 2010;64(3):371–7.

John R. Ward, MD: Pioneer— Clinical Trials in Rheumatology

H. James Williams, MD[1],*, Grant W. Cannon, MD[1],
Daniel O. Clegg, MD[1]

KEYWORDS

• Rheumatology • Controlled clinical trials • Outcome measures • Methotrexate

KEY POINTS

• Dr. Ward was an early pioneer in Rheumatology, especially in the intermountain West.
• Dr. Ward initially did basic research developing animal models of arthritis.
• Dr. Ward directed the CSSRD which completed important controlled clinical trials of treatments of rheumatic disease. The data was used to develop treatment response and remission criteria.

John Robert Ward was the founding father of rheumatology in the Intermountain West, the first Chief of the Division of Rheumatology at the University of Utah, and a national leader in the understanding and treatment of rheumatic disease. His foundational work established gold-standard techniques for the investigation of anti-rheumatic drugs. His leadership and scientific contributions clearly qualify him as a "giant in rheumatology" (**Fig. 1**).

BACKGROUND AND EDUCATION

Dr Ward was born on November 23, 1923, in Salt Lake City, Utah, the third of 7 children. Unfortunately, his family was left in impoverished circumstances due to his father's untimely death when he was just 10 years old. As the eldest son, Dr Ward said, "I became a kind of surrogate dad—more than I would have chosen."[1] He worked to help support his mother and 4 younger siblings. In fact, his mother was expecting his youngest brother at the time of his father's death.

Dr Ward attended primary and secondary public schools in Salt Lake City. Due to the ongoing strife from World War II, he enrolled at the University of Utah in a combined degree program. He was awarded a Bachelor of Science degree in 1944 and a Doctor

Division of Rheumatology, University of Utah School of Medicine, Salt Lake City, UT, USA
[1] Present address: 50 North Medical Drive, Salt Lake City, UT 84132, USA
* Corresponding author.
E-mail address: james.williams@hsc.utah.edu

Rheum Dis Clin N Am 50 (2024) 113–121
https://doi.org/10.1016/j.rdc.2023.08.009
0889-857X/24/© 2023 Elsevier Inc. All rights reserved.

rheumatic.theclinics.com

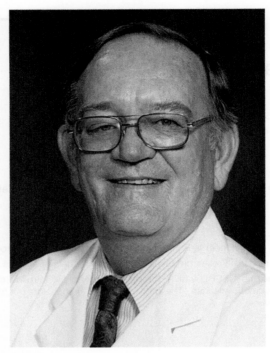

Fig. 1. John R. Ward M.D.

of Medicine degree in 1946. His class was the fourth class that had graduated from the University of Utah's newly accredited 4-year medical school. Following his graduation from medical school, Dr Ward became an intern, then resident, then chief resident at the Salt Lake County General Hospital, which was the teaching hospital for the University of Utah. He worked closely with his mentor, noted hematologist Maxw M. Wintrobe, MD, the first Chairman of Medicine at the University of Utah College of Medicine.

It was during this period that late one night, following a 48-hour shift as an intern, Dr Ward found himself in the nurses' dining hall, face-to-face with the evening nursing supervisor, Norma Harris. Romance blossomed, and Norma Harris and John R. Ward married in 1948, becoming life-long companions. Four children came from their union: John, Pamela, Scott, and James.

While a chief resident, Dr Ward was called to active duty in the Korean conflict where he served as Chief of the Medical Investigation Division at the Dugway Proving Grounds, US Army. Research, however, was Dr Ward's passion. "From the year I went into medical school, I wanted an academic career. Research seemed important, as well as seeing patients," said Dr Ward.[1] It was Dr Wintrobe's intent that Dr Ward become a hematologist. "I wasn't so eager about that," said Dr Ward. Subsequently, Dr Wintrobe extended the opportunity for future training to build Divisions in Gastroenterology, Infectious Disease, or Rheumatology within the Department of Medicine at the University of Utah. "This was about 1953. Cortisone had just been discovered, and it was very exciting. Rheumatology seemed like a challenging field at the time."[1] Therefore, after completing a research fellowship in physiology at the University of Utah, Dr Ward began a combined research and clinical fellowship at the Harvard Medical School along with the Massachusetts General Hospital focused on rheumatic diseases under the mentorship of Dr Walter Bauer. Dr Ward returned to the University of Utah College of Medicine as an Instructor of Medicine and Chief of the newly created Arthritis Division.

SCIENTIFIC CONTRIBUTIONS

While Dr Ward is primarily recognized for his foundational contributions in defining outcome measures and determining the effectiveness of early disease modifying medications in the treatment of inflammatory arthritis, he also established significant new methodologies and originated basic science concepts to advance fundamental understanding of rheumatic diseases (**Fig. 2**).

Basic Science Contributions

Dr Ward's contributions were principally in the investigation of potential infectious causes of rheumatic diseases and the development of animal models of arthritis. He was joined in this work by a basic science team that he recruited to the University of Utah, including Barry C. Cole, PhD; Marie M. Griffiths, PhD; and Leigh R. Washburn, PhD. When working with these Division of Rheumatology investigators and other collaborators in many areas of the School of Medicine at the University of Utah, Dr Ward provided remarkable insight into how investigations should be performed, offering valuable input for the successful implementation of their projects. These actions were not only productive scientifically but also facilitated his team in obtaining critical funding from both the National Institutes of Health and the Department of Veterans Affairs.

Infectious Agents in Rheumatic Diseases

The major focus of Dr Ward's basic science work was the evaluation of infectious agents considered to have the potential to produce rheumatic diseases. While he was involved in the study of the Newcastle virus and the rubella virus, the main concentration of his investigation was with Dr Barry C. Cole and Dr Leigh R. Washburn on *Mycoplasma* spp in animal models. While he did some limited work with *Mycoplasma pulmonis*, the majority of his research involved *Mycoplasma arthritidis*.[2,3] Using mouse, rat, rabbit, and even great ape models, his team described the clinical features of the *M arthritidis*-induced diseases in these animals. The pathology, pathophysiology, immunology, and genetics were therein successfully described.

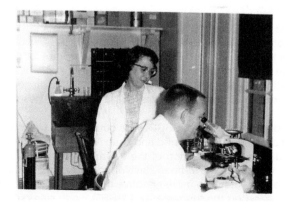

Fig. 2.

This work also led to the discovery of the *M arthritidis* mitogen, a superantigen identified in *M arthritidis* culture supernatant.[4] *M arthritidis* mitogen was shown to have significant immunologic activity and induced arthritis when injected into mice and rats. Leukocyte transformation assays were used to study the genetics of *M arthritidis* mitogen response in animal models, and the impact of in vitro anti-rheumatic drug effects on human lymphocytes.

Animal Models of Arthritis

Another major focus of Dr Ward's basic research was on animal models of arthritis. He accomplished some of the foundational work in adjuvant-induced arthritis, which is produced by the injection of Complete Freund's adjuvant into rats.[5] His work described the induction, histology, pathology, and immunology in these animals. The role of adjuvant-induced arthritis in the evaluation of anti-rheumatic drugs was also studied.

Dr Ward was involved in the evaluation of collagen-induced arthritis and the use of this model in the assessment of anti-rheumatic drug effects. The third animal model of arthritis evaluated by Dr Ward was 6-sulfanilaminoindazole-induced arthritis.[6] The effects of *M arthritidis* in this model and the genetic factors involved in susceptibility of rats to develop arthritis in response to 6-sulfanilaminoindazole were studied by Dr Ward's team.

In summary, Dr John R. Ward made significant contributions to basic science of rheumatic diseases through his individual work and through fostering and encouraging a productive research team of basic scientists that he recruited to the University of Utah. While no specific infectious agents associated with human rheumatic diseases were ever discovered by this work, his foundational research provided basic science understanding of some of the key models of arthritis, which have been used extensively by investigators throughout the world.

Clinical Studies in Rheumatology

In 1975, Dr Ward accelerated his efforts in clinical investigation while continuing his laboratory research. He and Mel Klauber, PhD, a biostatistician, applied for a contract with the National Institute of Arthritis and Musculoskeletal and Skin Diseases to establish a center to form a consortium of participating clinics with the expressed purpose of controlled clinical studies of rheumatic diseases. The contract was awarded to the University of Utah with the somewhat cumbersome name of the Cooperative Systematic Studies of Rheumatic Diseases (CSSRD). The coordinating center was at the University of Utah. Selected clinician investigators across the country were invited to participate in primarily placebo-controlled clinical studies in a number of carefully defined rheumatic diseases. The contract was renewed 3 successive times and the program lasted for nearly 2 decades (**Fig. 3**).

Dr Ward and Dr Klauber collaboratively directed the contract for the first year. When Dr Klauber left the University of Utah, Dr Ward became the sole director. He reorganized the coordinating center with James C. Reading, PhD, as associate director over data analysis and data storage and H. James Williams, MD, as associate director over clinical studies.

Most of the studies done by the CSSRD were comparative trials of treatments for a number of rheumatic diseases. The Food and Drug Administration (FDA) used some of these pivotal studies in the evaluation of the therapies for approval for clinical use. Over time, newer treatments have been developed and many of the agents studied have been replaced by safer and more effective treatments. Some current therapies, however, remain based on the fundamental CSSRD work, particularly methotrexate for rheumatoid arthritis. The pivotal controlled trial[7] of methotrexate versus placebo

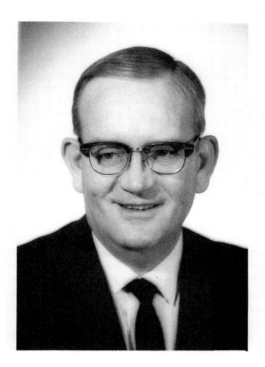

Fig. 3.

was used to gain FDA approval of this drug in the treatment of rheumatoid arthritis and provided critical information to support the broad implementation of methotrexate therapy in rheumatoid arthritis. Methotrexate has also now become the standard by which future therapies are measured. Methotrexate continues to be a foundational co-medication in disease-modifying anti-rheumatic drug (DMARD) trials.

The CSSRD provided a critical role in establishing the basis for all future DMARD clinical trials. The work of Dr Ward exhibited that large multicentered studies could be successfully conducted in patients with rheumatic disease. Results from these studies provided the essential foundational data for developing the currently employed measures for the evaluation of improvement such as the American College of Rheumatology 20% response criteria (ACR 20) and criteria for remission of disease activity.[8–10] Dr Ward was the motivating force behind most of the work done by the CSSRD. The CSSRD published 43 articles directly resulting from studies completed, and another 37 publications indirectly related to the CSSRD studies. Sixty-three abstracts were presented at scientific meetings.

MENTORSHIP

As mentioned earlier, Dr John R. Ward was the first and only rheumatologist in the Department of Medicine and in the state of Utah for many years. He was recognized as an outstanding clinician and an exceptional teacher among the students, residents, and fellows at the University of Utah School of Medicine (**Fig. 4**). The senior medical school clerkship in rheumatology was almost always fully subscribed. Medical students chose the elective to be able to work under Dr Ward and to learn from him. Similarly,

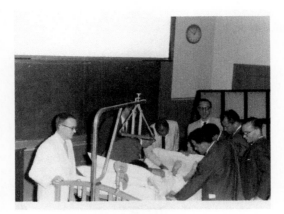

Fig. 4.

under Dr Ward, the rheumatology rotation among the internal medicine residents was very popular and fully subscribed. At the end of each rotation, Dr Ward haud a favorite and authentic Mexican restaurant where he would treat the students and residents. The mealtime conversation was animated and very memorable to all participants. When a fellowship in rheumatology was established, all of the fellows in the early years were graduates of the University of Utah School of Medicine and were influenced to enter the field of rheumatology because of Dr Ward's example of meticulous clinical care and compassion.

Dr Ward recruited one of these medical students, Cecil O. Samuelson, to train in rheumatology and join him on the faculty in the Division of Rheumatology. Dr Samuelson was trained in internal medicine and in rheumatology at Duke University and then returned to the University of Utah and joined Dr Ward as the second rheumatologist in the state of Utah. Dr Samuelson was mentored in the practice of rheumatology by Dr Ward and became a skilled clinician and was an outstanding teacher and academic administrator. Dr Samuelson subsequently became the Dean of the University of Utah School of Medicine, then Vice President of Health Sciences at the University of Utah. Dr Samuelson completed his academic career as President of the Brigham Young University.

Soon thereafter, Dr Ward recruited Dr H. James Williams to join the faculty. Dr Williams had also been a medical student at the University of Utah and had done his internal medicine postgraduate training at Duke University. He was strongly influenced to study rheumatology by Dr Ward, and was trained in rheumatology at the University of Utah, later joining Dr Ward and Dr Samuelson in the Division of Rheumatology. He developed a large practice and had a career in clinical investigation under the tutelage of Dr Ward. He was Associate Chairman of the Department of Internal Medicine for 26 years and succeeded Dr Ward as the Chief of the Division of Rheumatology. He was the second person from the University of Utah, after Dr Ward, to be selected as a Master of the American College of Rheumatology (ACR).

Dr Ward's third recruit to the Division of Rheumatology was Daniel O. Clegg, MD. He had been a medical student, intern, and resident at the University of Utah and was drawn toward rheumatology due to faculty interest and engagement. In fact, as a medical student working with Dr Ward and Dr Samuelson, he presented a paper at the national meetings of the ACR. Subsequently, Dr Clegg completed a fellowship in rheumatology at the University of Utah. He increased the visibility of rheumatology at the

George E. Wahlen Salt Lake City Veterans Affairs Medical Center (SLCVAMC), which became an essential part of the University of Utah teaching system. He saw patients at both the University and the SLCVAMC and was Chief of Rheumatology at the SLCVAMC. With Dr Ward's mentorship, Dr Clegg went on to develop large cooperative clinical trials in rheumatologic diseases through the Veterans Administration Cooperative Studies Program and the National Institutes of Health. He succeeded Dr Williams as the Division Chief and was the second of Dr Ward's protégés to be selected as a Master of the ACR.

It is remarkable that in 64 years, the Division of Rheumatology has had only three division chiefs. Dr Ward served from 1957 until 1990. Dr Williams served from 1990 until 1999, and Dr Clegg was Division Chief from 1999 until 2021. Dr Ward recruited and mentored both Dr Williams and Dr Clegg.

Dr Ward also recruited Grant W. Cannon to the Division of Rheumatology. Dr Cannon was Associate Chief of Staff for Education at the SLCVAMC from 1986 to 2020. Dr Cannon received his medical school, internal medicine, and rheumatology training at the University of Utah. He developed his own successful research and education programs at the SLCVAMC and became the third of Dr Ward's recruits selected to be a Master of the ACR.

Dr Ward recruited 3 other physicians to the Division before stepping down as the Division Chief. Two had not completed medical school at the University of Utah and one had been on a faculty of another institution. Dr Allen Sawitzke had been a house officer at the University of Utah followed by a fellowship in rheumatology under Dr Ward. He was a physician scholar and recipient of multiple teaching awards and served as Program Director for the fellowship. The other 2 remained on the faculty a few years before entering private practice in Salt Lake City.

During his tenure, the Division of Rheumatology at the University of Utah grew from a solo practice of 17 years to 7 rheumatologists. Dr Ward trained the majority of rheumatologists who entered private practice of rheumatology in Utah, Idaho, Nevada, and Montana. Other students became interested in rheumatology and trained at other institutions. Many of the later fellows came from without the state and, after finishing fellowship, went to practice in other areas of the country. It all began with Dr John R. Ward.

Dr Ward was also involved in mentoring trainees from other specialties including inter-disciplinary education of trainees from both the Department of Orthopedics and the Department of Physical Medicine and Rehabilitation.

PATIENT CARE

Dr Ward was an exceptional clinician. Across the medical school and in the community at large, patients who presented as diagnostic dilemmas were often referred for Dr Ward's opinion. As mentioned previously, Dr Ward brought rheumatology to the state of Utah. Not only was he the first and only rheumatologist in Utah for many years, he was the only rheumatologist between Denver and San Francisco and between Phoenix and the Canadian border. He provided specialty care in the rheumatic diseases for most of the Intermountain West.

In 1957, he founded and nurtured the Arthritis Division (later the Division of Rheumatology) in the Department of Internal Medicine at the University of Utah. Much later, in the 1970s, he recruited the first physicians who joined him in the Division. He established the fellowship program, which subsequently trained most of the rheumatologists who practiced in the Intermountain area over the subsequent decades. All physicians recognized him as the founding father of rheumatology in Utah (**Fig. 5**).

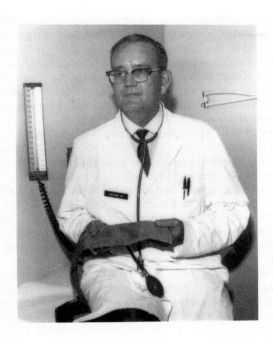

Fig. 5.

Dr Ward identified a lack of public health expertise in the School of Medicine and sought to find a solution. He was a member of the Utah Air National Guard and frequently flew to California in fulfillment of his duties. While continuing his work at the University of Utah, Dr Ward studied Public Health at the University of California and received his Master of Public Health from that institution. Following this training, Dr Ward was the founding Chairman of the Department of Preventive Medicine at the University of Utah. This department was the precursor for the Department of Family and Preventive Medicine, which is now the Department of Family and Community Medicine at the University of Utah.

His work as Director of the CSSRD for nearly 20 years helped to encourage controlled clinical trials. Studies were performed that helped increase understanding of the current therapies of rheumatic diseases.

With all of his academic responsibilities, he was always a popular and actively practicing rheumatologist. He saw patients from around the western United States. He was trusted and beloved by his patients, 2 of whom established academic chairs in rheumatology in his name.

IMPACT AND LEGACY

Dr Ward was one of the early academic rheumatologists in the nation and was the first and only rheumatologist in the state of Utah for many years, serving the entire Intermountain West. He established and nurtured the Division of Rheumatology at the University of Utah and instituted its expansion by inspiring University of Utah medical students, residents, and fellows to become academic rheumatologists.

His clinical skills and teaching abilities made the rheumatology elective particularly attractive to senior medical students. While most of the students interested in rheumatology did their fellowship at the University of Utah, some developed their interest from exposure to Dr Ward and then trained at other institutions before returning to Utah.

All 3 subsequent Masters of the ACR from the University of Utah consider Dr Ward their mentor.

Dr Ward was active in multiple leadership roles including committees of the University of Utah, American College of Physicians, ACR, Arthritis Foundation, National Institutes of Health, and FDA. He was recognized as an expert in the design and conduct of controlled clinical trials in rheumatology.

His work with the CSSRD, which compared treatment modalities, led to many publications. The data collected during CSSRD clinical trials were foundational for defining current disease activity measurements, functional assessments, and criteria for improvement and remission.

All this work was done while continuing to care for patients with rheumatic disease who recognized him as an exceptional physician and a compassionate friend.

DISCLOSURE

The authors have no commercial or financial conflicts and have no active funding sources.

REFERENCES

1. Sample S. Still Making a Difference–Tradition of Leadership, Patient Care Runs Deep in the Ward Family. Health Sciences Report University of Utah 2002;27(1):17–23.
2. Ward JR, Jones RS. The pathogenesis of mycoplasma (PPLO) arthritis in rats. Arthritis Rheum 1962;5:163–75.
3. Cole BC, Ward JR, Jones RS, et al. Chronic proliferative arthritis of mice induced by Mycoplasma arthritidis. I. Induction of disease and histopathological characteristics. Infect Immun 1971;4(4):344–55.
4. Cole BC, Washburn LR, Sullivan GJ, et al. Specificity of a mycoplasma mitogen for lymphocytes from human and various animal hosts. Infect Immun 1982;36(2): 662–6.
5. Ward JR, Jones RS. Studies on adjuvant-induced polyarthritis in rats. I. Adjuvant composition, route of injection, and removal of depot site. Arthritis Rheum 1962;5: 557–64.
6. Miller ML, Ward JR, Cole BC, et al. 6-sulfanilamidoindazole induced arthritis and periarthritis in rats. A new model of experimental inflammation. Arthritis Rheum 1970;13(3):222–35.
7. Williams HJ, Willkens RF, Samuelson CO Jr, et al. Comparison of low-dose oral pulse methotrexate and placebo in the treatment of rheumatoid arthritis. A controlled clinical trial. Arthritis Rheum 1985;28(7):721–30.
8. Paulus HE, Egger MJ, Ward JR, et al. Analysis of improvement in individual rheumatoid arthritis patients treated with disease-modifying antirheumatic drugs, based on the findings in patients treated with placebo. The Cooperative Systematic Studies of Rheumatic Diseases Group. Arthritis Rheum 1990;33(4):477–84.
9. Felson DT, Anderson JJ, Boers M, et al. The American College of Rheumatology preliminary core set of disease activity measures for rheumatoid arthritis clinical trials. The Committee on Outcome Measures in Rheumatoid Arthritis Clinical Trials. Arthritis Rheum 1993;36(6):729–40.
10. Williams HJ, Reading JC, Ward JR. Design and analysis of controlled clinical trials in rheumatic diseases. Clin Rheum Dis 1983;9(3):499–514.

The Giants of Rheumatology at Johns Hopkins: Lawrence E Shulman, MD, PhD and Mary Betty Stevens, MD

Marc C. Hochberg, MD, MPH, MACP, MACR

KEYWORDS

- Rheumatology • Systemic lupus erythematosus • Johns Hopkins

KEY POINTS

- Drs Lawrence E. Shulman and Mary Betty Stevens were the giants of rheumatology at Johns Hopkins during the latter half of the twentieth century.
- Together, they made immense contributions to our knowledge of systemic lupus erythematosus as well as other systemic autoimmune rheumatic diseases, and provided excellent clinical care to thousands of patients with rheumatoid arthritis, systemic lupus erythematosus, and other systemic autoimmune rheumatic diseases.
- Together, they trained almost 100 postdoctoral fellows, many of whom went on to highly successful careers in academic medicine, including the Directors of Divisions of Rheumatology and the Chairs of Departments of Medicine. Thus, their legacy was carried forward to the current generation of academic rheumatologists.

The history of rheumatology at The Johns Hopkins University School of Medicine and Medical Institution begins with Sir William Osler, the first Professor of Medicine in the School of Medicine and Physician-in-Chief of The Johns Hopkins Hospital who was appointed to these positions in 1889.[1] Among his many contributions to medicine, Osler largely is credited with the description of the visceral manifestations of systemic lupus erythematosus (SLE), based on systematic clinical observations of patients seen either on the wards of the Hospital or in the Medical Clinic, often with medical students and residents.[2] The sixth full-time Professor of Medicine, A McGehee Harvey solidified the reputation of Hopkins as a center for the study of SLE through his scholarly studies of this condition.[3] Dr Harvey established the Connective Tissue Division in 1955 and appointed Dr Lawrence E Shulman, then an Instructor in Medicine, as head. Thus begins our exploration of the contributions of the greats of Hopkins rheumatology, Drs

c/o Division of Rheumatology and Clinical Immunology, University of Maryland School of Medicine, 10 South Pine Street, MSTF 8-34, Baltimore, MD 21201, USA
E-mail addresses: mhochber@som.umaryland.edu; marc.hochberg@va.gov

Rheum Dis Clin N Am 50 (2024) 123–131
https://doi.org/10.1016/j.rdc.2023.08.010
0889-857X/24/Published by Elsevier Inc.

rheumatic.theclinics.com

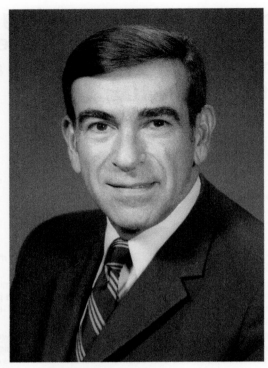

Fig. 1. Lawrence E Shulman, MD, PhD.

Lawrence E Shulman and Mary Betty Stevens, in the latter half of the twentieth century.

LAWRENCE E SHULMAN, MD, PhD

Lawrence (Larry) Edward Shulman was born on July 25, 1919, in Boston, MA, and raised in Brookline, MA (**Fig. 1**). He graduated from Boston Latin School; however, his schooling was interrupted for 1 year when he contracted polio. He matriculated at Harvard College and graduated in 1941. He spent the next 4 years working in the Department of Public Health under Prof Charles-Edward Amory Winslow at Yale University on projects related to the development of protective clothing for military troops operating in extreme cold and hot weather climates; this work was funded by the John B Pierce Foundation and resulted in a PhD in Public Health. Subsequently, he entered the Yale University School of Medicine and received his MD in 1949.

Larry came to Baltimore in 1949 and served as an intern on the Osler Medical Service at The Johns Hopkins Hospital. He later wrote that "This proved to be an unexpectedly exciting, exhilarating, educational and exhausting experience. … I became captivated with clinical medicine and have been ensnared thereby ever since."[4] Dr Harvey identified him as a unique young physician scientist and personally supervised his work on the effects of adrenocorticotrophic hormone (ACTH) and cortisone. Over the next 2 years, first as an Ayerst, McKenna and Harrison fellow in endocrinology, he pursued studies of ACTH and cortisone on hypersensitivity and then, as a Vernon D Lynch fellow, he studied the benefits and adverse effects of these agents in the collagen diseases, including SLE. He returned to complete his residency on the Osler Service and then joined the faculty of the School of Medicine as an instructor in Medicine in 1953. He was appointed to head the new Connective Tissue Division in 1955 by Dr Harvey and was promoted to the rank of Assistant Professor in 1956 and Associate Professor in 1964. Larry led the Division until 1975, the year before he left for the National Institutes of Health (NIH). I had the privilege and good fortune of being one of his last fellows, spending 6 months from July to December 1975 seeing patients with and learning from him in the Meyerhoff Private Outpatient Clinic and on the medical wards of The Johns Hopkins Hospital; we usually started daily inpatient consult rounds after 5:00 PM

Larry made seminal contributions to our knowledge of connective tissue diseases, particularly SLE and systemic sclerosis (scleroderma), his two main clinical interests. As a clinical research fellow, he worked with Dr Harvey as well as Drs Philip Tumulty, C Lockard Conley, and Edith H Schoenrich on the seminal Hopkins paper based on a careful analysis of 138 cases of SLE[3]; I am pleased to have a copy of the bound reprint of this paper, personally signed by Dr Harvey and given to me before I left Hopkins in 1991. Dr Shulman was the first to apply the life-table method to study the prognosis of patients with SLE; they reported that the 4-year cumulative survival was only 51% in this cohort of patients.[5] During this time, he also worked with Dr Joseph E Moore and helped establish the relationship between the presence of a chronic biologic false-positive test for syphilis and possible, probable, or definite SLE as well as other connective tissue diseases in almost half of such patients.[6]

Dr Shulman mentored the clinical research careers of several postdoctoral fellows focused on SLE; two of note were Dr Mary Betty Stevens, a postdoctoral fellow from 1958 to 1960, and Dr Frank C Arnett, Jr, a postdoctoral fellow from 1970 to 1972. Dr Stevens' work with Dr Shulman will be discussed below; herein, I will briefly comment on the work of Dr Arnett with Dr Shulman to analyze the familial occurrence of SLE. They reported eight families and analyzed 53 cases in 25 families in total.[7] They noted a strong concordance for disease manifestations in identical twin pairs and parent-offspring pairs but not in sib pairs, supporting a genetic contribution to the etiology of SLE. These studies laid the groundwork for Dr Arnett's career as a physician–scientist in rheumatology not only at Hopkins but also at the University of Texas Health Sciences Center in Houston where he was the Director of the Division of Rheumatology, the Chair of the Department of Medicine, and the first Director of the Center for Clinical and Translational Sciences before his retirement.

Dr Shulman's other major clinical interest during his tenure at Hopkins was systemic sclerosis (scleroderma). He and his fellows, Drs William D'Angelo and James Fries, and his colleague, Alphonse Masi, wrote a seminal paper on the pathologic findings in systemic sclerosis comparing autopsies in 58 cases that had died in Baltimore area hospitals between 1948 and 1966 and age, sex, race, and hospital-matched controls.[8] They reported that autopsied cases had more pulmonary involvement, both interstitial fibrosis and pulmonary arteriolar thickening; myocardial fibrosis, particularly in younger patients; coronary arteriolar lesions, fibrinous pericarditis, muscle atrophy, and/or fibrosis in all areas of the gastrointestinal tract; and renal arteriolar disease, similar to that seen in patients with malignant hypertension. Dr Rida Frayha and other postdoctoral fellows worked with him to report the frequency and type of hematologic abnormalities and cranial nerve involvement, most often a sensory trigeminal neuropathy, in large series of patients with systemic sclerosis seen at Hopkins.[9,10]

Because of this clinical interest and his renown as an excellent physician, he was the recipient of many referrals of patients with connective tissue diseases. Of particular relevance, were two men with a scleroderma-like illness characterized by firm taught skin over the arms and legs but sparing the hands accompanied by peripheral eosinophilia, elevated erythrocyte sedimentation rate, and hypergammaglobulinemia who had striking thickening of the fascia between the subcutis and muscle on full-thickness biopsies. These patients were initially presented at the VIth Pan-American Congress of Rheumatology in 1974 and along with two additional cases, published in 1975.[11] I actually saw one of the latter two patients, Case 4 in this article, with Dr Shulman in the Meyerhoff outpatient clinic during my fellowship.

In 1978, Fu and colleagues described four additional cases and summarized 23 cases reported since Dr Shulman's original paper and coined the eponym "Shulman's syndrome" for the syndrome of eosinophilic fasciitis characterized by eight features (**Box 1**).[12] Dr Shulman commented on these and other subsequent cases and noted that the pathogenesis of eosinophilic fasciitis remained obscure.[13] Later, he compared and contrasted the clinical and laboratory features of eosinophilia-myalgia syndrome and toxic oil syndrome with eosinophilic fasciitis and noted that some patients initially diagnosed with eosinophilia-myalgia syndrome subsequently developed the full picture of eosinophilic fasciitis.[14]

Dr Shulman spent 20 years as the Director of the Connective Tissue Division at Hopkins before transitioning to the next phase of his career at the NIH. The list of postdoctoral fellows that he trained at Hopkins who went on to noteworthy and successful careers in academic medicine includes, but is not limited to, Drs Mary Betty Stevens, Alexander S Townes, Murray Urowitz, James F Fries, Bevra H Hahn, Frank C Arnett, Graciela S Alarcon, and myself.

Dr Shulman was appointed as the first Associate Director for Arthritis, Musculoskeletal and Skin Diseases at the National Institute of Arthritis, Metabolism and Digestive Diseases in 1976. He was named the Director of the Division of Arthritis, Musculoskeletal and Skin Diseases at the National Institute of Arthritis, Diabetes, Digestive and Kidney Diseases in 1983 and was the inaugural Director of the National Institute of Arthritis and Musculoskeletal and Skin Diseases when it was formed in 1986. He retired from NIH on October 1, 1994, at the age of 75 years. Following his retirement, the late Dr J Claude Bennett wrote the following regarding his tenure at the NIH: "In his scientific leadership role, Larry has demonstrated the utmost commitment not only to advancing our understanding of the pathogenetic, diagnostic, therapeutic, and rehabilitative aspects of these diseases but also to rapidly and effectively transferring

---

Box 1
Features of Shulman's syndrome[10]

- Rapid onset
- Recent history of exertion
- Sclerodermoid skin changes
- Absence of Raynaud's phenomenon and visceral involvement of progressive systemic sclerosis
- Hypergammaglobulinemia G
- Peripheral blood eosinophilia
- Histologically nonspecific inflammatory reaction involving fascia, with extension into the adjacent muscle and subcutaneous tissues
- Dramatic response to systemic prednisone therapy

useful knowledge directly to practicing physicians, to patients and their families, and to voluntary health organizations and other lay and professional groups championing the cause of general or specific medical research."[15]

Dr Shulman was the President of the American Rheumatism Association (now American College of Rheumatology [ACR]) from 1974 to 1975 and the President of the Pan American League of Associations of Rheumatology from 1982 to 1986. He received numerous honors during his career; the two that he was most proud of were the Heberden Medal in 1975 and the Presidential Gold Medal from the ACR in 1996. Dr Shulman passed away in 2009 from bladder cancer; he is survived by his daughters Kathy Shulman and Barbara Shulman-Kirwin and grandchildren. Dr Bevra H Hahn wrote that "The world of rheumatology has lost a great man. We miss him, honor him, and continue to draw inspiration from him."[16]

MARY BETTY STEVENS, MD

Mary Betty Stevens was born on January 11, 1929, in Cambridge, New York, and raised in Granville, a small town in upstate New York bordering Vermont (**Fig. 2**). She matriculated at Vassar College and graduated in 1948. After 1 year as a teaching assistant at Mount Holyoke College, she came to Baltimore in 1949 with plans to become a research scientist and served as an Assistant in Chemistry at the School of Hygiene and Public Health before deciding to matriculate at the School of Medicine in 1951. She received her MD in 1955 and completed her internship and residency on

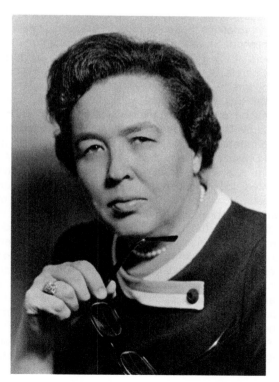

Fig. 2. Mary Betty Stevens, MD. (Hahn BH: In memoriam: Mary Betty Stevens, MD, FACP, FACR, 1929-1994. Arthritis Rheum 1995;38:444.)

the Osler Medical Service from 1955 to 1958 and postdoctoral fellowship in the Connective Tissue Division from 1958 to 1960.

Mary Betty joined the faculty of the School of Medicine as an instructor in Medicine in 1960. She rose through the faculty ranks, eventually being named Professor of Medicine, and remained on the faculty until her death in 1994.

As a fellow and junior faculty member, Mary Betty worked with Dr Shulman on clinical research studies in patients with lupus and other connective tissue diseases, including the importance of the finding of extracellular material on LE cell preparations and the association between esophageal dysmotility and Raynaud phenomenon.[17,18] As an Assistant Professor, she became the Director of the Hopkins Outpatient Arthritis Clinic and implemented nurse management programs for patients with rheumatoid arthritis receiving intramuscular gold injections and patients with gout receiving prophylactic colchicine and urate-lowering therapy. During this time, she also developed her remarkable bedside teaching skills which were recognized when she received the George J Stuart Award for best clinical teacher from the Hopkins' graduating class of 1971. Ted Rose, President of the class, stated "A lot of people are brilliant in their field, but they can't seem to get their thoughts across. Dr. Stevens manages both, and at the same time she shows great concern for the students."

In 1970, Dr Stevens was appointed as the Director, Division of Rheumatology and Head of a new 36-bed inpatient Rheumatic Disease Unit (RDU) at the Good Samaritan Hospital. In this position, she pioneered the multidisciplinary team approach to the care of patients with rheumatoid arthritis and other rheumatic diseases involving orthopedic surgery, physical and occupational therapy, social work, nursing, and nutrition in addition to rheumatology. Serving as a subintern on this unit became one of the most popular elective rotations for senior medical students almost immediately after the RDU was established. Several of my classmates and I completed this elective; indeed, five members of my graduating class of 1973 (Drs David Borenstein, Marc Hochberg, Joseph Scarola, Stuart Silverman, and Dennis Torretti) became rheumatologists. I spent 6 months of my first year of fellowship from January to June 1976 covering the inpatient RDU, alternating call with either the Hopkins or Maryland Senior Resident and learning on rounds and at the bedside from not only Dr Stevens but also Drs Frank Arnett, Carole Dorsch, Abdullah Shams, and Thomas Zizic.

Dr Stevens was promoted to Associate Professor and appointed as the Director of the newly renamed Division of Rheumatology in 1975 by Dr Victor A McKusick, succeeding Dr Shulman. She was the first woman to become the Division Director in the Department of Medicine at Hopkins. In the same year, she was named the Director of the Division of Rheumatology at the University of Maryland School of Medicine by Dr Theodore Woodword; this provided an unique opportunity for the amalgamation of clinical teaching of medical students and residents from both academic institutions in Baltimore under one combined faculty. During this period, under her leadership, the inpatient RDU and the outpatient practice at Good Samaritan Hospital developed an international reputation for multidisciplinary patient care and training of not only rheumatology fellows but also arthritis-related health professionals, including nurses and physical therapists. She was assisted in these latter efforts by Ms Joan D Sutton, a clinical nurse specialist in rheumatology who held faculty appointments at both the School of Medicine and School of Nursing until her death in 1991.[19]

Dr Stevens supervised original clinical research in SLE by her postdoctoral fellows and faculty colleagues including descriptions of central nervous system involvement, ischemic necrosis of bone, abdominal vasculitis and colonic perforation, ocular involvement, and a comprehensive summary of racial/ethnic and sex/gender differences in 150 patients with SLE.[20–27] She also supervised original clinical research in other systemic autoimmune rheumatic diseases, including polymyositis, rheumatoid arthritis, and Sjogren syndrome, among others that resulted in a total of more than 50 peer-reviewed publications.

Dr Stevens stepped down as the Director of the Division of Rheumatology at the University of Maryland in 1985 and at Johns Hopkins in 1987 but remained the Director of the RDU until her death in 1994. The list of postdoctoral fellows whom she trained who went on to successful careers in rheumatology includes, but is not limited to, Drs Thomas M. Zizic, David Borenstein, Dennis Torretti, Frederick Wigley, Joan Bathon, and myself.

Dr Stevens was the Second Vice-President, American Rheumatism Association (now ACR) and elected as Master of both the ACR and American College of Physicians. She received numerous honors during her career; the two that she was most proud of were the George J Stuart Award (vide supra) and the Distinguished Rheumatologist Award from the ACR in 1990. Dr Stevens passed away in 1994 from complications of a stroke. Dr Bevra H Hahn wrote that "Dr. Stevens was unfailingly enthusiastic about teaching, patient care, and the creation of new information. She inspired patients, students, residents, fellows, and colleagues to reach higher, to push back the barriers of our limited knowledge, to excel. She was the ultimate role model and mentor."[28]

PERSONAL REFLECTIONS

I was fortunate to have been a student and fellow under both Drs. Shulman and Stevens during my training at Johns Hopkins. As mentioned above, I completed the subinternship on the inpatient RDU at Good Samaritan Hospital during my senior year and got to witness first-hand the excellent patient care delivered by Dr Stevens and was the recipient of her bedside teaching. I particularly recall watching her sit on the edge of a patient's bed to discuss their symptoms, diagnosis, and treatment, a unique bedside manner that I continue to emulate when I make consult rounds with our fellows.

I spent the first half of my first year of fellowship working with Dr Shulman at Hopkins covering the inpatient consult service and seeing his patients in the private outpatient clinic. The second half was spent on the inpatient RDU working with Dr Stevens and her colleagues. During my second year, after Dr Shulman had transitioned to his new position at the NIH, he came to dinner at our apartment and charted my future career path with the recommendation that I obtain formal training in epidemiology to become a researcher in public health. When I approached Dr Stevens with this idea, she agreed to support me as a part-time student at the School of Hygiene and Public Health when I joined the faculty as an instructor in Medicine. I then spent 2 years studying for an MPH while working half-time seeing outpatients and attending on the RDU and covering the inpatient consult service at Hopkins.

I owe the success of my career to their combined mentorship that continued as I rose through the faculty ranks at Hopkins before leaving to join the faculty at the University of Maryland. The current internationally recognized rheumatology division at Hopkins stands on the shoulders of these giants.

DISCLOSURE

The author has no potential conflicts of interest to disclose.

ACKNOWLEDGMENTS

The author wishes to thank Ms Terri L Hatfield, MLIS, Reference Archivist, Alan Mason Chesney Medical Archives, Johns Hopkins Medicine, Nursing and Public Health, for access to papers and photographs related to both Dr Lawrence E Shulman and Mary Betty Stevens. The portraits of both Drs Shulman and Stevens are reproduced from images included in the archives.

REFERENCES

1. Harvey AM, McKusick VA, Stobo JD. Osler's legacy: the Department of Medicine at Johns Hopkins 1889-1989. Baltimore, MD: The Department of Medicine, The Johns Hopkins University; 1990. p. 1–18. Chapter 1.
2. Hochberg MC. The history of lupus erythematosus. Md Med J 1991;40(10): 871–3.
3. Harvey AM, Shulman LE, Tumulty PA, et al. Systemic lupus erythematosus: review of the literature and clinical analysis of 138 cases. Medicine (Baltim) 1954;33(4): 291–437.
4. Shulman R: Some personal highlights of Lawrence E. Shulman's life. In Hahn BH, Arnett FC, Zizic TM, Hochberg MC, editors. Current Topics in Rheumatology: A collection from Johns Hopkins Fellows, Past and Present. 1983, xiii-xv.
5. Merrell M, Shulman LE. Determination of prognosis in chronic disease, illustrated by systemic lupus erythematosus. J Chron Dis 1955;1:12–32.
6. Moore JE, Shulman LE, Scott JT. The natural history of systemic lupus erythematosus: an approach to its study through chronic biologic false positive reactors; interim report. J Chron Dis 1957;5:282–9.
7. Arnett FC, Shulman LE. Studies in familial systemic lupus erythematosus. Medicine 1976;55:313–22.
8. D'Angelo WA, Fries JF, Masi AT, et al. Pathologic observations in systemic sclerosis (scleroderma): a study of fifty-eight autopsy cases and fifty-eight matched controls. Am J Med 1969;46:428–40.
9. Frayha RA, Shulman LE, Stevens MB. Hematological abnormalities in scleroderma: a study of 180 cases. Acta Haematol 1980;64:25–30.
10. Teasdale RD, Frayha RA, Shulman LE. Cranial nerve involvement is systemic sclerosis (scleroderma): a report of 10 cases. Medicine (Baltim) 1980;59:149–59.
11. Shulman LE. Diffuse fasciitis with eosinophilia: a new syndrome? Trans Assoc Am Physicians 1985;88:70–86.
12. Fu TS, Soltani K, Sorensen LB, et al. Eosinophilic fasciitis. JAMA 1978;240:451–3.
13. Shulman LE. Diffuse fasciitis with hypergammaglobulinemia and eosinophilia: a new syndrome? J Rheumatol 1984;11:569–70.
14. Shulman LE. The eosinophilia-myalgia syndrome associated with ingestion of L-tryptophan. Arthritis Rheum 1990;33:913–7.
15. Bennett JC. A tribute to leadership: Lawrence E. Shulman, MD, PhD, and the National Institute of Arthritis and Musculoskeletal and Skin Diseases. Arthritis Rheum 1994;37:1577.
16. Hahn BH. In memoriam: Lawrence E Shulman, MD, PhD, 1919-2009. Arthritis Rheum 2010;62:311.
17. Stevens MB, Abbey H, Shulman LE. The clinical significance of extracellular material (ECM) in LE cell preparations: I. Analysis at the time of the first abnormal test. N Engl J Med 1963;268:976–82.
18. Stevens MB, Hookman P, Siegel CJ, et al. Aperistalsis of the esophagus in patients with connective tissue diseases and Raynaud phenomenon. N Engl J Med 1964;270:1218–22.
19. Stevens MD. In memoriam: Joan D. Sutton, RN, MSN. Arthritis Care Res 1992; 5:57–8.

20. Feinglass EJ, Arnett FC, Dorsch CA, et al. Neuropsychiatric manifestations of systemic lupus erythematosus: diagnosis, clinical spectrum, and relationship to other features of the disease. Medicine (Baltim) 1976;55:323–39.
21. Klipper AR, Zizic TM, Stevens MB, et al. Ischemic necrosis of bone in systemic lupus erythematosus. Medicine (Baltim) 1976;55:251–7.
22. Zizic TM, Hungerford DS, Stevens MB. Ischemic necrosis of bone in systemic lupus erythematosus: II. The early diagnosis of ischemic necrosis of bone. Medicine (Baltim) 1980;59:134–42.
23. Zizic TM, Shulman LE, Stevens MB. Colonic perforations in systemic lupus erythematosus. Medicine (Baltim) 1975;54:411–26.
24. Zizic TM, Classen JM, Stevens MB. Acute abdominal complications of systemic lupus erythematosus and polyarteritis nodosa. Am J Med 1982;73:525–31.
25. Jabs DA, Fine SL, Hochberg MC, et al. Severe retino-occlusive disease in systemic lupus erythematosus. Arch Ophthalmol 1986;104:558–63.
26. Jabs DA, Miller NR, Newman SA, et al. Optic neuropathy in systemic lupus erythematosus. Arch Ophthalmol 1986;104:564–8.
27. Hochberg MC, Boyd RE, Ahearn JM, et al. Systemic lupus erythematosus: a review of clinico-laboratory features and immunogenetic markers in 150 patients with emphasis on demographic subsets. Medicine (Baltim) 1985;64:285–95.
28. Hahn BH. In memoriam: Mary Betty Stevens, MD, FACP, FACR, 1929-1994. Arthritis Rheum 1995;38:444.

Hal Holman of Stanford

William Neal Roberts Jr[a],*, Edward R. Lew, BA[b],
Matthew H. Liang, MD, MPH[c,d]

KEYWORDS

- Hal Holman • Clinical scholars program • Systemic lupus • Stanford

KEY POINTS

- Social activist as a student, as a laboratory scientist, physician, and medical leader.
- Demonstrated the autoimmune basis of systemic lupus erythematosus.
- Developed new models of education for clinician scientists in the Robert Wood Johnson Clinical Scholars Program.

INTRODUCTION

Born in 1925, Holman came of age at a time of enormous changes in society and medicine. **Figs. 1–3** Abraham Flexner's report on *Medical Education in the United States and Canada* (a.k.a. the Flexner Report) had exposed the deplorable quality of medical education, thereby precipitating the closure of the majority of medical schools.[1,2] The First World War and its aftermath laid the ground for the next conflagration. The Great Depression galvanized new leaders who promised relief. In the Second World War, 70 million people perished. Those returning home were determined to make the most of the opportunities presented to them and to get on with their lives, as society was committed to helping them. The War ended the depression, brought women and African-Americans into the work force, assisted military veterans to obtain higher learning through the GI Bill, and started the military-industrial complex and the Veterans Administration Health care system.

This account is based on *Halsted R. Holman and the Struggle for the Soul of Medicine*[3] and focuses on Holman's legacy in rheumatic disease—namely, his discovery at the Rockefeller Institute, which pioneered the understanding of systemic lupus erythematosus (SLE) as an auto-immune disease of unknown etiology—as well as his legacy in medical education, social justice, and the Robert Wood Johnson (RWJ) Clinical Scholars.

[a] Division of Rheumatology, University of Kentucky Medical Center, Lexington, KY, USA;
[b] Department of Political Science and Legal Studies, University of Massachusetts Amherst, 150 South Huntington Avenue, Boston, MA 02130, USA; [c] Rheumatology Section, Jamaica Plain VA Medical Center, 150 South Huntington Avenue, Boston, MA 02130, USA; [d] Division of Rheumatology, Inflammation, and Immunity, Brigham and Women's Hospital, Boston, MA, USA
* Corresponding author. Rheumatology, 740 South Limestone, J511 Lexington, KY 40536.
E-mail address: neal.roberts@uky.edu

Rheum Dis Clin N Am 50 (2024) 133–146
https://doi.org/10.1016/j.rdc.2023.08.011
0889-857X/24/© 2023 Elsevier Inc. All rights reserved.

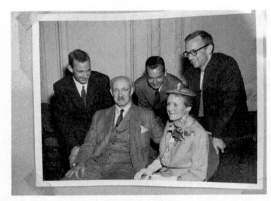

Fig. 1. Ann and Emile Holman with their adult children. Hal is in the center. [Source: Holman family scrap book]

The Early Days

As a second-generation immigrant, Holman had models of social conscience from his parents, both of whom were physicians and fierce believers in doing what was right even if it meant flaunting convention. His father, Emile Frederic Holman, was the son of a Methodist minister. His family had fled Bismarck's Germany to California before the First World War. Emile graduated from Johns Hopkins Medical School and was the last Chief Resident at Hopkins under William Stuart Halsted and Mont

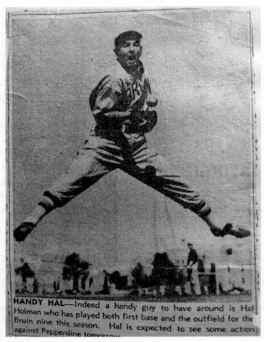

HANDY HAL—Indeed a handy guy to have around is Hal Holman who has played both first base and the outfield for the Bruin nine this season. Hal is expected to see some action against Pepperdine tomorrow.

Fig. 2. Scrapbook newspaper clipping of Holman in UCLA baseball uniform with "Bruins" legible on the jersey. In addition to batting .506 "Handy Hal" was apparently an agile fielder. [Source: unknown but likely from UCLA student newspaper 1944 or 1945]

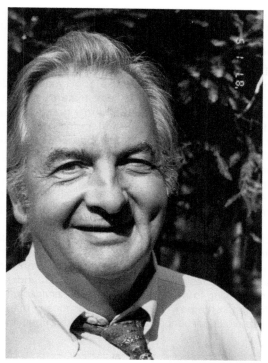

Fig. 3. Portrait photograph, Hal Holman at Stanford in 1987. [Source: Holman family scrap book].

Rogers Reid; Halsted Reid Holman was named after them. In 1923, Emile worked under Dr. Harvey Cushing at Peter Bent Brigham Hospital. He was recruited to Stanford at age 36 and chaired the Department of Surgery until he was 66. His observations of grafting skin from a mother to a severely burned child laid the groundwork for modern burn management.

Halsted's mother, Ann Peril Purdy, was from a Canadian farm family. She was the only person in her family to attend college. Ann Purdy graduated from McGill in 1915 followed by Johns Hopkins. She was one of the first female graduates of both universities. At Johns Hopkins, she met and married Emile. Ann was a clinical professor of pediatrics and saw largely pediatric cardiology patients, almost 30 years before the formal beginning of the specialty.

In 1943, Halsted registered for the draft, like all men his age, and volunteered for the Navy's program to accelerate medical training to ensure enough doctors for the Second World War. Two courses changed Halsted's world view as a freshman at Stanford: Biology inspired him to become a physician and a required course on the History of Western Civilization introduced him to Karl Marx's philosophy.

The Navy sent him to the University of California Los Angeles (UCLA) for his second and last year as an undergraduate. Holman was a good student and a first-string halfback on the varsity team, until he separated his shoulder. Bobby Brown, future cardiologist and Yankee third baseman on 4 World Series championships, recruited Holman to shag balls with him. By year's end, he was batting an astounding 0.506

and an UCLA All-Star. The Chicago White Sox and San Francisco Seals minor league tried to entice him into professional baseball, but he wanted to be a doctor.

Yale Medical School and International Advocacy

After 1 year at UCLA, the Navy sent Holman to Yale Medical School. After his second year, he received a fellowship in biochemistry and took a year off to do basic research. He was elected to the Alpha Omega Alpha society. In the Yale library, he met Barbara Lucas studying public health. She had been an Army nurse, caring for quadriplegic soldiers returning from the Second World War, after graduating from Bryn Mawr College in philosophy. She was deeply moved by how one's positive attitude could affect the survival of soldiers with severe war injuries.

Holman and other Yale students revived the Association of Interns and Medical Students (AIMS) chapter. The chapter combated racism through a Yale–Meharry exchange program. A few months after joining, he resigned from the Communist Party so as to not compromise AIMS. Holman was elected president of the national organization.

After medical school, Holman was selected for a National Research Council Fellowship in Biochemistry at the Carlsberg Laboratories in Copenhagen. Holman agreed to represent AIMS in the International Union of Students (IUS) in Prague. Its president was Joza Grohman, a fierce resistance fighter of the Czech underground during the Second World War. Traveling to improve student health services gave Holman a close look at events unfolding in the provision of health services in many European countries. That experience would influence his thinking about population health care.

Persona Non Grata

In 1950, Senator Joseph McCarthy's search for the "enemies from within" occupied the news for the next 4 years. Prominent cultural and social leaders testified before his committee about their knowledge of the communist conspiracy. From 1951 to 1955, the Federal Bureau of Investigation (FBI) distributed anonymous files alleging Communist affiliations of citizens, opened mail, performed illegal wiretaps, and "subterfuges" in the Counterintelligence Program to discredit political organizations. Holman was under surveillance during his house staff training in the Bronx and was questioned by agents about Americans he had known in Europe.

By 1950, the State Department decided that American youth abroad should not be working in organizations like the IUS, which worked in socialist-bloc countries. Holman was asked by the American Embassy in Denmark to relinquish his passport. He ignored the order and moved with Barbara to Prague, where he worked full-time for the IUS. In 1951, he was ready to return to Yale to continue his medical training. With the confiscation of his passport always looming, Holman and Barbara reentered the United States by a freighter in Athens bound for Canada and entered the United States by train. In New Haven, he was offered an internship from John Peters, Chairman of the Department of Medicine, in July 1952.

After returning to San Francisco to see his family, Holman got a call from Peters, "You better come back here—they're trying to take your internship away from you." Holman returned to New Haven and learned that if he wanted to keep his internship, he would have to sign a loyalty oath. He had been a member of the Communist Party for only a few months before he resigned, but he strongly objected to the oath as an intrusion of government into the views of its citizens. Peters could not have been more sympathetic to Holman but let the process play itself out. Holman met with members of an Executive Committee who would decide his fate. The first person expressed his appreciation of Holman and his political activities but ultimately capitulated under pressure: "I have to be candid with you," he said. "I'm going to vote against you, and the reason is: I'm afraid. If I don't, they may turn their attention to me."

Another interviewer was Gustav Lindskog, Chairman of Surgery and a former Navy lieutenant commander, who said to Holman, "I really hate you. I hate everything you stand for. I think what you've been doing is disreputable, and I have zero sympathy for the causes you favor. However, they have absolutely no right to take away an internship because of your political positions—and so, despite what I think about you, I'm going to vote for you." A few days later, the Executive Committee voted to expel Holman.

Montefiore Hospital

Losing his internship at Yale, Holman had to find a place for house staff training. Bernard Lown (1921–2021), who had first met Holman as a Yale house staff, was now at Montefiore and told the Department of Medicine that Holman might be available. Holman warned Montefiore officials that he would not sign the loyalty oath. Despite that, they offered him a position. Those events of hiring an academic star from an Ivy League school, who had been dismissed from his internship, to a hospital with strong Jewish roots must be appreciated in the context of the world between 1938 and the beginning of the Second World War. Anti-Semitism was prevalent in many American hospital training programs and medical schools.

Located in northwest Bronx—a working class area with many Catholic, Protestant, and Jewish families from Europe—it began in 1884 as the Montefiore Home for Chronic Invalids for the care of those whom other hospitals would not help. Its Jewish physicians understood what it was like to be mistreated for one's beliefs and had a reputation for hiring those blacklisted during the McCarthy era. The hospital had carved out a special place in American medicine. It accepted the first female intern in 1916, African-American residents in the 1930s, and had one of the first residencies in social medicine in the country.

Before he started training, Holman was summoned before the Subcommittee of the Senate Judiciary Committee probing *Communist Tactics in Controlling Youth Organizations* in US student organizations. At the hearing, Holman's effort to receive counsel was constantly interrupted. Two-thirds of the way through the meeting, his lawyer, Marshall Perlin, was ordered to leave because of "contemptuous behavior." The Subcommittee grilled Holman about his involvement with AIMS, the IUS, and Americans he had met in Europe. The hearing never amounted to much and Holman started his internship without further incident.

Holman was an intern, Assistant Resident in Medicine, and Chief Resident in Neoplastic Diseases at Montefiore. During his residency, he received a Korean War Doctors Draft notice twice, ignored the loyalty oath each time, and was deferred twice to complete his residency. A third final notice was for immediate induction. He refused to sign the loyalty oath but was inducted anyway. However, Holman developed tuberculosis and was treated at the Montefiore Sanitarium for 3 months and his induction postponed for 5 years automatically. By then, the Korean War was over, his residency was completed, and the Doctors' Draft ultimately declared unconstitutional.

Rockefeller University Hospital

In 1910, the Rockefeller Hospital opened America's first 30-bed inpatient unit where persons with diseases of interest were admitted and studied. When Holman arrived at the Rockefeller, 6 of the eventual 24 scientists associated with the university had already won the Nobel Prize.

For instance, working in Henry Kunkel's Lab with him were Edward C. Franklin (1928–1982) and Hans Müller-Eberhard (1927–1998). They shared authorship on one study of the relationship between the high molecular weight (19S) and low molecular weight (7S) antibodies and the nature of the autoantibody-like factor, rheumatoid factor, seen in patients with rheumatoid arthritis (RA).

Franklin, the first author, and his family had fled Nazi Germany. He was the only child of a prosperous Berlin lawyer and his wife. Franklin's family waited until late 1938, perhaps reflecting the ambivalence that well-established Jews felt about leaving their homeland. In the United States, Franklin graduated from high school at age 15, cum laude in biochemistry from Harvard at age 18, and received his MD from New York University. After house staff training at New York's Beth Israel Hospital and Montefiore, military duty and residency at Bronx Veterans Administration Hospital, he found a "cauldron of excitement" with "endless stimulating discussions at all hours of the day or night." Kunkel's enthusiasm for the then recently published work on antibodies and myeloma drew Franklin to those areas. Almost a third of Franklin's publications dealt with γ-globulins, or as they would ultimately be called, the immunoglobulins.

Han's father, Adolph Müller, a successful businessman in Germany, changed his family name to Müller-Eberhard after the Second World War to memorialize his son who was killed on the Russian front at age 21. His father was fervently against Nazism and warned Hans to not tell others about his views on Hitler, lest he be sent to a concentration camp. Hans was the only member of his class not to join the Hitler youth. At age 17, Hans was drafted and sent to Hungary. Toward the close of the war, he was captured by the Russians. He managed to escape by hiding in a ditch during the day and traveling by night through forests. He ultimately reached the Danube, was captured by United States forces, and eventually rejoined his family in Altenau, Germany, where he began schooling. His teacher, Fritz Hartmann, had visited Henry Kunkel in New York who suggested that Hartmann might send his students to work at the Rockefeller as postdoctoral trainees. Emerging from war-torn Germany, Müller-Eberhard found there an "effervescent" community of young and old scholars.

Discovering the Autoimmune Basis of Systemic Lupus Erythematosus

In the early 1900s, Paul Ehrlich was studying isoantibodies to red blood cells and concluded that autoantibodies directed against the host cells or their constituents, did not occur. He believed that autoimmunity, if it did exist, could be fatal and coined the term "horror autotoxicus."

This view persisted despite the emerging evidence of autoreactivity in diseases such as sympathetic ophthalmia and thrombocytopenic purpura. The explicit recognition of autoimmunity did not occur until a new generation (trained in genetics, biology, and in various medical subspecialties) joined the mainstream of immunology.

In 1948, Hargraves, Richmond, and Morton described the lupus erythematosus (LE) cell phenomena in the bone marrow of certain patients.[4,5] They had observed a neutrophil or macrophage in what appeared to be engulfing nuclear material from the breakdown of other cells. This phenomenon was seen in persons with systemic lupus erythematosus (SLE) and other rheumatic disorders, and only after their blood had been at room temperature. The cell became a diagnostic criterion for lupus, but what caused the phenomenon was a mystery.

Within a few years, Haserick, Lewis, and Bortz showed that in lupus, the gamma globulin fraction of blood stimulated production of LE cells. When gamma globulin levels fell during clinical remissions, the LE cells also disappeared from the blood.[6] Miescher and Fauconnet[7] mixed serum from lupus patients with crushed cell nuclei and the nuclear material used up the specific gamma globulin and prevented the formation of the LE cell.

In 1957, alone in the laboratory at night, Holman had his eureka moment. He isolated the serum factor that adhered to cell nuclei and showed that the separated antibody was absorbed by another preparation of nucleoprotein. Nucleoprotein is the main constituent of chromosomes which are deoxyribose nucleic acid (DNA) and histone. Exposing phagocytes to the antibody-coated nucleoprotein, he also showed that the cells quickly engulfed the material producing the LE cell thus completing the explanation and proving that the LE cell phenomena resulted from a reaction between the patient's own immune globulin and the DNA of the patient's chromosomes.[8,9]

Holman wanted to present his work at the prestigious meeting of the American Society for Clinical Investigation, but Kunkel felt the work was not ready for submission. Holman felt differently and asked Jules Hirsch, a Rockefeller colleague who had just been inducted into the Society, to sponsor the abstract. It was selected for the Plenary Session, traditionally the showcase of the most important work of the meeting. Holman's presentation was warmly received; Kunkel seemed surprised but was still unsure of its importance. He urged Holman to present his findings to Elvin Kabat, a protein chemist and thought leader. Holman succeeded in convincing Kabat that the protein he had identified was, indeed, an antibody gamma globulin engaged in an immune reaction with the DNA part of the DNA-histone complex and was responsible for the LE cell phenomena. The 1200-word discovery was published in *Science*[8] and provided definitive proof of autoimmunity in SLE.

Holman's work and that of others from that period has been somewhat lost in accounts of autoimmunity or of the search for the pathogenesis of SLE,[10–17] except for one.[18] In science, discoveries may be made simultaneously and independently by more than one person or group.[19] Others build on previous work or work by individuals. A scientist may not have realized its own work's significance or recognized a discovery as such. Forgetting and selective memory occur in science just as it does in daily life. It is seen when a scientist leaves a field as was the case with Holman. Science does not necessarily progress in a linear fashion, but after one generation is replaced by younger scientists unconstrained by existing scientific paradigms.[20]

An autoantibody to DNA in SLE is demonstrated in Holman's landmark paper.[8] It describes the antecedent work of Miescher and Fauconnet[7] and also cites Friou's "similar observation."[21–23] Ultimately, Friou's fluorescent antinuclear antibody detection, based on the Coombs technique, became a diagnostic test for lupus. What was most important was that it engaged a generation of scientists pursuing immunologic mechanisms in new concept of pathogenesis.

Over time, Holman changed his thinking about the role of autoimmunity in SLE and had concerns about where his work had taken the field. He had begun working in the 1950s with the concept of autoimmunity that had an acute phase marked by disease-specific auto-antibodies such as anti-nuclear antibody (ANA), anti-ribonuclear protein (RNP) and mixed connective tissue disease (MCTD). However, antinuclear antibodies could not explain SLE's varied organ manifestations, and the path to specific treatment remained uncertain. He had seen many individuals misdiagnosed and mismanaged because they had a positive ANA. He came to the view of autoimmunity as a normal response and that autoantibodies can often be found in normal people. Those with SLE may have an exaggerated response.[24]

Holman's view moved toward a new model of chronic diseases evolving over time in a matrix of interactive soluble, cellular, and social factors. He gently described this hypothesis in a 1994 editorial as an argument for a biopsychosocial synthesis of disease.[25] He felt that assuming a single pathway might disappoint and that clinical observations on various clinical phenotypes and individual responses should not be ignored but incorporated. Emphasis on initial events might be replaced by a model in which the acute phase of initiation of autoimmune disease was superseded by a longer phase. During the chronic phase, the disease evolves away from the initial events toward even more complex interaction happening within a multi-pathway matrix. This matrix consisted of humoral elements easy to purify and work with in the lab; different linages of cells which were harder to isolate, classify, and study; and finally, in the big picture, social factors—impossible to purify or to single out. In this big matrix, zip codes can dominate genetic codes.

Holman took this view into the trenches of patient care, experimental design, clinical research, and education. He remained an experimentalist but also embraced and challenged the unwieldiness of the social factors in the matrix with creative, clever, and sometimes inspired experimental designs and outcome measures.

Building the New Stanford Medical Center

Holman's journey back to California occurred during a tumultuous time. From 1960 to 1969, similar cultural and political trends occurred all around the world. The United States, United Kingdom, France, Italy, and West Germany turned to the political left and 34 African countries gained independence from their European rulers. Worldwide, wars and internal violence marked the era: Vietnam War, Bay of Pigs Invasion, Portuguese Colonial War, Indo–Pakistani War, Arab–Israeli Six Days War; internal violence in Nigeria, Laos, Sudan, People's Republic of China, Northern Ireland, France, Mexico and coup d'états in Greece, Iraq, and Libya. In the United States: assassinations of Malcolm X, John F. Kennedy, Martin Luther King Jr., and Robert Kennedy; police assaults on innocent protesters at the 1968 Democratic National Convention; the Compton's Cafeteria Riot; and the Stonewall Riots. The Civil Rights movement mobilized thousands of college students.

Following the Second World War, the country invested heavily in science and medicine, rapidly expanded the National Institutes of Health (NIH) and research at academic medical centers. Between 1965 and 1990, the full-time medical faculty increased more than 4-fold; NIH funding increased 11-fold; and revenues of academic medical centers increased by providing treatment from Medicare and Medicaid; moreover, revenues of the health insurance industry increased nearly 200-fold.

For Stanford, the sea changes in funding came at a propitious moment. What had begun in 1908 as the Cooper Medical College in San Francisco became the Stanford University School of Medicine in Palo Alto in 1959. In moving, Stanford built a new facility and faculty from scratch. Holman was also on the short list of other institutions.

A letter from Henry Kunkel to Joshua Lederberg—the year before Lederberg won the Nobel Prize in Medicine and Physiology—recommended Stanford consider Holman for a larger role than an Associate Professorship. That led to an endowed chair as Chairperson of the Department of Medicine. At age 35, he became the youngest Department of Medicine Chairperson that Stanford (and possibly any medical school) ever had. The FBI was still pestering Holman and tried to block his appointment, calling him a dangerous subversive.

Holman set out to recruit faculty who shared his enthusiasm for biomedicine. These cutting-edge thinkers were young and excelled at both clinical medicine and laboratory science. He started a model cross-department research collaboration that became a hallmark of the new immunology and a magnet for other like-minded faculty. The first new Division that Holman created at Stanford was Immunology and Rheumatology. He was his only faculty until 1966, when Hugh McDevitt (1930–2022) was recruited. As a Harvard medical student, he did not know what he was going to do, but a rotation at the Robert B. Brigham and a stint in a lab showed him a path in the biosciences. Jim Fries (1938–2021), Sam Strober (1940–2022), Gary Fathman, Ted Pincus, PJ Utz, and Mark Genovese joined the group eventually.

Educational Philosophy

Given the license and freedom to set the educational thrust of the new enterprise at Stanford, Holman's philosophy had been heavily shaped by watching his mother ministering to patients in their home, in college struggling in a course, and his readings on educational philosophy, as well as the hospitalized SLE patients at the Rockefeller. At UCLA, Holman was lost in a Greek philosophy course until the instructor gave a 3-page summary of what problems the philosophers were addressing. Only after this did he had the understanding to decipher the various ruminations covered in the course.

He was inspired by Paolo Freire whose *Pedagogy of the Oppressed*[26] had just been translated into English. It drew on Freire's success helping Brazilian adults read and write. Strongly influenced by Karl Marx, Freire felt that traditional teaching treated students as empty vessels to be filled with knowledge, thereby oppressing both student and teacher. He argued that education should help people be more fully human and treat learners as co-creators of knowledge. Freire believed that true freedom resulted from informed action when a balance between theory and practice was achieved.

Holman's other inspiration was Evans Carlson who led the "Carlson's Raiders" of the Second World War in the Pacific. The son of a minister, Carlson had run away from home and lied about his age to enlist in the First World War. A year after discharge, he enlisted in the Marines. In 1937 to 1938, he was a military observer of Mao Zedong, Zhou Enlai, and Deng Xiaoping in northern China where he learned their guerrilla tactics against the Japanese. When Carlson took command of the Second Marine Raider Battalion, the military divided officers and enlistees in a caste system. His experience in China had convinced him of a better model: Leaders served the unit, and fighters on the ground planned the next battle. The soldiers were led but also served.

At the Rockefeller, Holman cared for patients who had difficult refractory disease and/or were unable to pay for medical care. Caring for lupus patients there left a lasting impression on his approach. Patients remained in the hospital for at least a month and received free medical care and private tutors if they were in school. Many patients were terrified about their disease when first admitted, but as they learned more about what was known and not known, they grew calmer. Holman gave patients his home telephone number with instructions to call with questions, day or night, so they wouldn't have to deal with physicians who were not familiar with their care. The patients rarely called, and then only for truly urgent questions. Holman learned the importance of educating patients about their disease and developed a deep respect for their resilience and that they would find the way, even when the prognosis was uncertain or grim.

In medical and postgraduate education, Holman was skeptical of theoretic or academic solutions that were implemented before they were tested in real life. He strived to stimulate and encourage the full creativity of the learner into solving important problems and urged that the process be egalitarian, collaborative, and inclusive. All of this came together in his work with the RWJ Clinical Scholars.

The Robert Wood Johnson Clinical Scholars Program

In the 1960s, many criticized education as being dominated by white, male, western views. Basic education was felt to be 2 systems: one for people who became employees and the other for people who became the leaders. In medical education, there was a perception that the technical aspects of medicine were crowding out the humanistic care and that health disparities were growing.

The idea for the Clinical Scholars program began in 1969, at a meeting in Swampscott, Massachusetts, addressing the future of medical education and patient care needs.[27] At lunch, Holman, John Beck from McGill, Julius Krevans from Johns Hopkins, Austin Weisberger from Case Western, and Jim Wyngaarden from Duke thought they could improve the sensitivity of medical care to its patients. It would be accomplished by changing medical education to produce a new kind of physician with a strong grasp of the societal forces that impact health care, the quantitative and qualitative skills to assess these forces and the health care system, and the ability to effect change within the system. The Carnegie Corporation and the Commonwealth Fund launched the Clinical Scholars Program. In 1971, the program was transferred to the RWJ Foundation.

In 1971, Stanford Medical School appointed a new Dean: Clayton Rich. Holman offered his resignation pro forma believing that a dean should have the right to appoint department chairs. It gave the University the perfect opportunity to oust him. Holman felt that his politics might have played a role, but it wasn't all: "I think the basic motivation was that I was not sufficiently clinically oriented and that we needed to strengthen our clinical work as opposed to our bioscience. A lot of people, I think, felt that way."

Tom Merigan and other colleagues felt otherwise: "Holman was always a clinician. He got his research materials from his patients and was always involved in their care. He was involved with ensuring clinical excellence, a theme he continues to this day."

By the time he resigned, Holman had already shifted his focus. He made the case in his Presidential address, "Sounds from a Different Drum," to the American Society for Clinical Research.[28] He poured his energies into the new Clinical Scholars Program from 1969 to 1996, and then formed the joint Stanford–the University of California, San Francisco (UCSF) Clinical Scholar program with Julius Krevans as the Program Director at the UCSF.

The Program had a distinct west coast, laid-back style. It had no theme and no curriculum. Each Scholar's "program" was individually developed. To be selected, the applicant had to convince Holman and others that they were pursuing something important; that they were capable of doing it or had a plan for acquiring the tools. The supervision was permissive at best, adopting the operating principle of the "freedom to fail." Holman encouraged Scholars in "action research" where one implements an intervention (action) and evaluates it in a real-life setting (research).

The Scholars program was a hot bed of ideas in a time of social unrest. New thinking and writings dominated their discussions and conferences. Although Holman was immersed in mechanistic laboratory experiments, he was also a student of psychology, sociology, economics, history, political theory, philosophy—anything that would help him understand the many factors influencing health and what could be done. The major literature all appeared in a 10-year period.

In *Medical Nemesis*,[29] Illich argued that one's health was too important to be left to the professional; the patient needed to be involved. Health, he wrote, is the capacity to cope with the human reality of death, pain, and sickness. Technology can help, but modern medicine has gone too far into a battle to eradicate death, pain, and sickness. In doing so, it turns people into consumers or objects, destroying their capacity for health.

Cochrane[30] showed that many medical and surgical practices have had little critical evaluation. Thomas McKeown's *The Role of Medicine*[31] challenged the belief that finding the cause and the specific treatment of a disease would lead to health, the biomedical medicine premise. He pointed out that tuberculosis, rheumatic fever, and diphtheria had already become less prevalent by the time the specific microbial agent and specific antibiotic were discovered. He also felt that "the major threat to health in the world [was] modern medicine," and what medical students saw in venerable teaching hospitals was more for the benefit of doctors than patients. Medicine had become commodified, bureaucratic, more business than a calling.

Amos Tversky and Daniel Kahneman described the heuristics and biases employed when people are faced with making choices under uncertainty.[32] Their impact on many areas of science and medical decision-making was profound and was recognized in a Nobel Prize to Kahneman in 2002; by then, Tversky had passed away of metastatic melanoma at age 59 at Stanford.

Victor Fuchs' *Who Shall Live?*[33] applied ideas in economic theory to medical care in a way that had not been done before and was credited with kick-starting the field of health economics. The book presented the challenges in allocating health resources efficiently and equitably, and he identified the 3 major problems with US health care: high cost, gaps in access, and inferior measures of population health.

In 1995, funding for the Stanford–UCSF program was not renewed following Holman's retirement. The reason for the decision was never clear. The rest of the Clinical Scholars Programs ended in 2017. Many problems that preoccupied Scholars were being appropriated within medical and surgical specialties or by people in managerial sciences, quality assurance activities, implementation sciences, and for-profit management consultants—all done full-time, often by non-clinicians, or for profit.

The RWJ Clinical Scholars had an extraordinary run. Some 20% of former Scholars became leaders in health care organizations, hospitals, medical schools, and public health—e.g., the Institute of Medicine, the Health Resources and Services Administration, the National Institute of Health, Health and Human Services, the Communicable Disease Center, state and city public health departments. Six deans of schools of public health, as well as Surgeon General David Satcher, had been Scholars.

Over the years, 65 went through the Stanford–UCSF program. Jim Fries was the first Clinical Scholar at Stanford. He was described as a dashing, mustached, charismatic figure, climber of the 6 highest peaks on 6 continents, marathon runner, plane pilot, equestrian, who drove a red convertible. Fries created the Arthritis, Rheumatism, and Aging Medical Information System, a national computerized arthritis database for tracking outcomes in SLE, RA, and later stroke and human immunodeficiency virus. Its functionality foretold the electronic medical record, data mining, and "patient learning systems" many years later.[34,35] With John Ware, Bob Meenan, Lawren Daltroy, Lewis Kazis, Matt Liang, Chris Murray and others, they expanded the measurement of function in many conditions and argued that function was an essential vital sign like height, weight, blood pressure, pulse rate, and respiratory rate to describe a person's state and a population health metric. This happened long before Congress authorized the Patient-Centered Outcomes Research Institute in 2010 and made patient-oriented outcomes a field in itself.

In rheumatic and musculoskeletal conditions especially, the Scholars Program was an incubator of health services and health policy research, clinical epidemiology, and outcomes research: Holman, Wallace Epstein, Fries, Robert Meenan, Matthew Liang, Mike Ward, Stan Shoor; Rick Deyo, Claire Bombardier were just some of the clinician scientists who led the way.

Personal Impact

Halsted R. Holman is arguably one of the century's great leaders who led by doing, changing, responding to the challenges of the times, and inspired a generation to action and a view they could barely perceive. At a peace rally in the Bronx, Holman met Clarence B. Jones who eventually was to become a civil rights lawyer and confidante to Martin Luther King. Jones was completely taken by Holman, who "looked like William Holden" and once described him as "a man for all seasons." The Montefiore medical house staff seemed in awe of him. At Holman's 19th birthday, celebration and symposium at Stanford, there was an outpouring of affection for him, a long list of people who wanted to speak. For many there that day, he had touched a part of their soul. Several attendees quipped it was like "returning to Camelot." During a break, they clamored to hear more from him.

As a young Chief of a new enterprise and new faculty at Stanford where there was little age difference between its leaders and the trainees, Holman felt led to a rich social network of peers: "We not only did laboratory work together and saw patients together, but we went out together, played sports together" and "the rigid, hierarchical life that was classical for academia just dissolved here, and we liked it that way."

He expresses tremendous personal warmth, particularly with people from whom he stands to gain nothing; and at Stanford he seemed always above the fray. Each Clinical Scholar felt they had a special relationship with him. They referred to him as "silver-tongue" in awe of his eloquence, optimism, and principles. He hated pretense, the cult of the celebrity, the arrogance of the "excellence deception," and was a sponge for knowledge from the range of human thinking.

Words matter a great deal to him and getting it right was a way we learned about thinking deeply and communicating ideas. He recognizes that technical jargon can be divisive, elitist, and get in the way of understanding. In the Clinical Scholars program, he probed for the simplest explanation so that every participant would feel comfortable. There was no such thing as a final draft. He had a talent for translating what one was trying to communicate in a way that contextualized its importance, made it better, bigger, grander, and helped them find their voice.

A modest, eloquent person, with a looming presence, athletic grace, a baritone orator's cadence in a button-down shirt, his sleeves are usually rolled up. When teaching at Stanford, his arms were filled with annotated xerox copies of scholarly journals and monographs that he might have encountered in the New York Review of Books to share. Lecturing and writing left-handed, sparingly on the blackboard, he made difficult things simple and simple things nuanced. His arguments were clear and connected emotionally; the audience was often spell-bound. In 1975, Senator Ted Kennedy chaired a public debate on recombinant DNA organized by Dr. Larry Horowitz who was also a Stanford Clinical Scholar. Horowitz remembers the senator leaning back and whispering in his ear on 2 occasions as Holman spoke before the spotlights: "He should run for office!" "He should just record this on vinyl [records]!"

DISCLOSURE

None.

FUNDING

None.

REFERENCES

1. Flexner A. Medical education in the United States and Canada: a report to the carnegie foundation for the advancement of teaching. 1910.

2. Franklin E, Holman HR, Müller-Eberhard HJ, Kunkel HG. An unusual protein component of high molecular weight in the serum of certain patients with rheumatoid arthritis. J Exp Med 1957;105:425–38.
3. Liang MH, Lew ER, Halsted R. Holman and the struggle for the soul of medicine. Newcastle upon Tyne, England: Cambridge Scholars Publishing; 2022.
4. Hargraves MM, Richmond Helen, Robert J. Morton. Presentation of Two Bone Marrow Elements: The 'Tart' Cell and the 'L. E.' Cell. Proc Staff Meet Mayo Clin 1948;23(2):25–8.
5. Hargraves MM, Richmond Helen, Robert J. Morton. Production in Vitro of the L.E. Cell Phenomenon: Use of Normal Bone Marrow Elements and Blood Plasma From Patients With Acute Disseminated Lupus Erythematosus. Proc Staff Meet Mayo Clin 1949;24(9):234–7.
6. Haserick J, Lewis Lena, Bortz Donald. Blood Factor in Acute Disseminated Lupus Erythematosus 1. Determination of Gamma Globulin as Specific Plasma Fraction. Am J Med Sci 1950;219(6):660–3.
7. Miescher P, Fauconnet ML. 'absorption du facteur L.E. par des noyaux cellulaires isolés. Absorption of L.E. Factor by Isolated Cell Nuclei. Experientia 1954;10:252–4.
8. Holman HR, Kunkel HG. Affinity Between the Lupus Erythematosus Serum Factor and Cell Nuclei and Nucleoprotein. Science 1957;126(3265):162–3.
9. Holman HR. Report Concerning a Mid-Peninsula Cooperative Health Maintenance Organization. 1974. https://searchworks.stanford.edu/view/12430343.
10. Hahn BH. Antibodies to DNA. N Engl J Med 1998;338(19):1359–68.
11. Isenberg DA, Manson JJ, Ehrenstein MR, et al. Fifty Years of Anti-ds DNA Antibodies: Are We Approaching Journey's End? Rheumatology 2007;46(7):1052–6.
12. Kumar Y, Bhatia A, Minz RW. Antinuclear Antibodies and Their Detection Methods in Diagnosis of Connective Tissue Diseases: A Journey Revisited. Diagn Pathol 2009;4(1):1–10.
13. Mahler M, Meroni P-L, Bossuyt X, et al. Current Concepts and Future Directions for the Assessment of Autoantibodies to Cellular Antigens Referred to as Anti-Nuclear Antibodies. Journal of Immunology Research 2014;2014(315179):1–18.
14. Plotz PH. Autoimmunity: The History of an Idea. Arthritis Rheumatol 2014;66(11):2915–20.
15. Silverstein AM. A history of immunology. 2nd edition. Cambridge, MA: Academic Press; 2009.
16. Silverstein AM. Autoimmunity *Versus Horror Autotoxicus*: The Struggle for Recognition. Nat Immunol 2001;2(4):279–81.
17. Tsokos GC. Systemic Lupus Erythematosus. N Engl J Med 2011;365(22):2110–21.
18. Anderson W, Mackay IR. Intolerant bodies: a short history of autoimmunity. Baltimore, MD: Johns Hopkins University Press; 2014.
19. Gladwell M. In the air. New York, NY: The New Yorker; 2008.
20. Kuhn TS. The structure of scientific revolutions. Chicago, IL: University of Chicago Press; 1962.
21. Friou GJ, Finch SC, Detre KD, et al. Interaction of Nuclei and Globulin from Lupus Erythematosis Serum Demonstrated with Fluorescent Antibody. J Immunol 1958;80(4):324–9.
22. Friou GJ, Finch SC, Detre KD. Nuclear localization of a factor from disseminated lupus serum. presented at: Federation Proceedings; 1957; Available at: https://archive.org/details/DTIC_AD0634942/page/n15/mode/2up.

23. Friou GJ. The Significance of the Lupus Globulin-Nucleoprotein Reaction. Ann Intern Med 1958;49(4):866–75.

24. Holman HR. Systemic Lupus Erythematosus: Disease of an Unusual Immunologic Responsiveness? Am J Med 1959;27(4):525–8.

25. Holman HR. Thought Barriers to Understanding Rheumatic Diseases. Arthritis Rheum 1994;37(11):1565–72.

26. Freire P. Pedagogy of the oppressed. Ramos MB. Continuum; 1970.

27. Gardner JR, Krevans J, Mahoney M. A Conversation about the Clinical Scholars Program: The Training of Nonbiomedical Fellows inside the Modern Academic Medical Center. Medical Care 2002;40(4):25–31. Supplement: A Festschrift in Honor of Halsted R. Holman, M.D.: Action Research in Health Care):II25–II31.

28. Holman HR. Sounds From a Different Drum. J Clin Invest 1971;50(6):1369–72.

29. Illich I. Medical Nemesis: the expropriation of health. New York, NY: Pantheon Books; 1975.

30. Cochrane A. Effectiveness and efficiency: random reflections on health services. London, UK: Nuffield Trust; 1972.

31. McKeown T. The role of medicine: dream, mirage or Nemesis? London, UK: Nuffield Trust; 1976.

32. Tversky A, Kahneman D. Judgment Under Uncertainty: Heuristics and Biases. Science 1974;185(4157):1124–31.

33. Fuchs VR. Who Shall live? Health, economics, and social choice. New York, NY: Basic Books; 1975.

34. Fries JF, Holman HR. Systemic lupus erythematosus: a clinical analysis. Philadelphia, PA: W.B. Saunders; 1975.

35. Fries JF. A Data Bank for the Clinician? N Engl J Med 1976;294(25):1400–2.

Printed and bound by CPI Group (UK) Ltd, Croydon, CR0 4YY

08/05/2025

01864748-0007